Think
yourself
FIT

Think yourself
FIT

Gloria Thomas

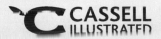
CASSELL
ILLUSTRATED

First published in Great Britain in 2003 by
Cassell Illustrated, a division of
Octopus Publishing Group Limited
2-4 Heron Quays, London E14 4JP

A CIP catalogue record for this book is available
from the British Library.

ISBN 1 84403 011 3

Design and illustrations by Tanya Devonshire-Jones
Photography by Bill Norton

Printed in Italy

DEDICATION

I would like to dedicate *Think Yourself Fit* to
my son Jamie Thomas and the next generation
of potential fitness enthusiasts. I really hope
that you can apply this new way of thinking
to your lives and your children's lives so that we
become a fitter, more active nation and physical
fitness simply becomes a part of everyday life.

*Disclaimer – It is advisable to consult a physician
in all matters relating to health and in particular to
check with your doctor before embarking on any
exercise regime. While the advice and information
in this book is believed to be accurate and true at
the time of going to press, neither the authors nor
the publisher can accept any legal responsibility or
liability for any injury sustained whilst following
the exercises.*

Contents

Introduction

We are constantly being told that obesity is becoming more normal as a large percentage of the population is completely inactive. How have we allowed ourselves to become this way? The answer to this lies in the way we respond to the world around us, our attitude to life, the decisions we make and the actions that we take.

The result of this conditioning is that we have learned to rely on external resources to take us to where we want to go in life. If you consider how many fitness books, exercise videos, gadgets and health clubs there are that are supposed to encourage healthy lifestyles you would think the whole world would be active. Certainly, we are clearer about what we need to do with regard to exercise but somehow there are many of us who just don't do it. Amazingly, with all the incredible amount of knowledge around us we seem to have avoided the 'how to' at a most crucial level. We have ignored the mental and emotional aspect of exercise.

With the emergence of new ways of thinking that enable us to explore our experience by tapping into the resources of the mind we can reset the balance by working in a more empowered way. We all have the ability to do so much more than we think we can. We just have to find out how. You can learn to become more skilled mentally which will result in a more motivated and positive attitude to exercise, health and your life. Through these pages you will learn a new approach that will teach you simple ways to make a difference to the way you think. You can get up and get moving, you can enjoy getting more active and you can be more consistent in your exercise regime if you want to. This book enables you to explore your current mind set and shows how to make changes where needed.

Now it is time now for you to help yourself and focus on the tools that will enable you to get fit from the inside out as well as the outside in. I hope this book is useful to you.

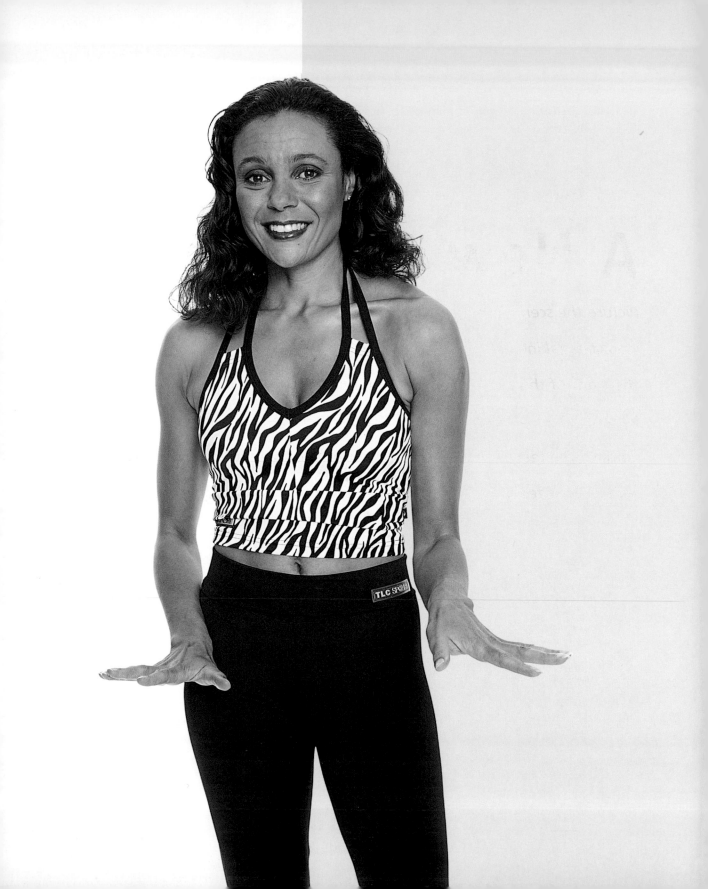

Chapter 1

A New Attitude

Picture the scene. A bright studio with a well-sprung wooden floor. A step class taking place with me (the person whose picture you see on the front of this book) limbering up for some action. Now add some vibrant, driving Latino sounds and the rather masculine monotone voice of the teacher booming out instructions for the class to follow. Add a bit of feeling to this picture – excitement and apprehension.

A New Attitude

I'm really looking forward to the lovely music but these types of classes have a tendency to be very choreographed, and in truth I like simple high-intensity classes. A voice begins to start nagging at me, 'You know you can never follow these complicated routines, what on earth are you doing?' The music is in full swing and the teacher begins the main part of the class. 'Step on the box, step off it – up, up, down, down – now lead with the other foot – good, you've got it – now do an open turn and step over the box.' So far, so good, but as I continue to listen to the instructor I begin to feel a little anxious, and the inner voice starts again: 'She's going to make the routine really complicated and there's no way that you'll be able to follow it.'

As I listen to this inner dialogue my concentration is no longer on the class. And while I've been distracted, the teacher has put in some new moves. Tricky ones too. When I bring my attention back to her I am lost. I seem to have two left feet and shoot off in the wrong direction. 'You stupid idiot,' the voice yells at me. 'I told you so.' Tense and anxious, I'm worrying too much about the footwork. I was so looking forward to moving to the Latino music. To save face and keep going I start to do my own thing – a simple samba, a basic step, a few star jumps. Yes, that should raise my heart rate and my esteem again. In the mirror I catch a glimpse of the teacher scowling at me. Oh no! She's annoyed because I'm not following her routine. The negative self-talk starts again. 'Call yourself a fitness professional? You can't even follow a routine.' Sheepishly I revert back to the instructor's moves so that I don't offend her. But I've lost track of the routine completely. I have no idea where I am going now and I promptly trip over the step. My own words have become a self-fulfilling prophecy. I have proven myself right: I can't follow the class. I leave the studio feeling deflated and frustrated. 'I won't be going back there again.'

We talk to ourselves all the time although we are rarely aware of it. Sometimes the talk is constructive and positive. But more often than not it is the opposite: critical, harsh and counter-productive.The way we use language both internally and externally affects the way that we think and the actions we take. Most of this self-talk is learned from experiences we have had. Even new experiences have associations with old ones in order that we can make sense of what is happening around us. Therefore the inner dialogue that is going on today is mainly the product of past experience.

My Experience

I started to take my fitness seriously at the age of 13 when I dreamed of running the 200 metres for England. I was good at sport. At school I was frequently called up in assembly to be presented with medals and certificates for achievements in hockey and athletics, and I even made the all-England trials for long jump. There was nothing more important to me in life than running. Even if I close my eyes now I can remember the feeling of excitement, a great sense of freedom and elation as I ran. A confidence that whatever I turned my hand to in life I would achieve. But a virulent strain of glandular fever and a number of other events in my life shattered that dream. After what seemed a long period off from school, and sapped of my energy and strength, I no longer had the physical or mental resources to participate seriously in the sport I loved. It was then that the negative inner dialogue began, and I became well practised at talking myself out of any potentially challenging or tiring situation. This negative self-talk began to guide me in every area of my life.

Your mind works just like a computer. It is capable of doing just about anything within reason that it is programmed to do. One of the functions of the inner mind is to house the imagination. When you are young your imagination encourages you to achieve your dreams and make them a reality. What happens to our younger selves and the input of family, friends and teachers interact with the imagination and have a direct affect on how we experience the world around us – for better or worse. The experiences of childhood can influence the way we think for the rest of our lives. Mine would burden me for more than ten years.

I became active again at the age of 28. I was suffering from a bout of post-natal depression after a fairly traumatic childbirth. My son came prematurely into the world by emergency Caesarean. He was very poorly and had difficulty breathing. Because I looked fit and well I was discharged within days of the birth and had to commute to the hospital to feed my son. It was exhausting having to take a bus to and from the hospital twice a day after such a major operation, but it was all worth it when my son came home fighting fit one month later. Soon after this traumatic event, I decided, as do many women of today, to go back to work and combine motherhood with a career. I was offered a job as a presenter on cable television. I was exhausted by motherhood and hadn't allowed myself to recover fully from the birth. I was also inexperienced, anxious and uncertain of my abilities. Negative self-talk seemed to haunt me relentlessly, reinforcing my already limiting beliefs about my self and my capabilities. My contract ended 18 months later and I withdrew from the world.

We are thinking machines that never shut down. We take in information from the world around us: everything we have ever seen, heard, felt, smelled, tasted is stored inside our computer-like minds to be called on when needed. The more often we repeat a thought or a

The words that we repeat to ourselves, day in day out, become our reality.

suggestion the more deeply ingrained in our mind it becomes. As time goes by and our characters form and develop, the words that we repeat to ourselves, day in day out, become our 'reality'. The thoughts and suggestions of everyday life have, through repetition, formed the map of the world we live in.

I decided that I had to do something to help myself and I started to explore ways to move away from this low state of mind. My first thoughts were of the positive associations that I had of the sports field. I took myself off to the local athletics track. Even though I was extremely unfit and felt extremely silly trailing in behind everyone else, the experience of becoming active again was wonderful. I felt the familiar exhilaration and feelings of well-being that physical exertion brings. Shortly after my return to the athletics track I went on a family holiday to St Lucia. As I was lying on the beach, meditating on life in general, I became aware of some activity not far away: an aerobics class. I was fascinated as I watched the teacher doing her stuff. And I knew that I could do the same too. It would give me the confidence to face the world. It would help me feel better and I would get fighting fit. My mind was made up. I now had a focus for the future.

Although I didn't realize it, this was probably one of the most positive decisions I had made in my life. Even if the negative self-talk continued, especially at the prospect of me teaching aerobics, I was determined to do something for myself. I wanted to find the way forward. When I got home I made enquiries and signed up for a course on exercise instruction. And it was with knees knocking and my voice a little weak and an incredible sense of pride that I stood, a qualified instructor, in front of my first class.

Although we are the products of our conditioning we can make changes in our lives if we choose to. Conversely, if we always do what we have always done we will always get what we have always got in the past. The longer we hold on to negative thoughts and actions, the harder it is to change them. To change our actions we need to change our thinking. The first step forward is to want whole-heartedly to change and to know that you can make that change happen. You then become curious to find the right way forward for you. And when you direct your thoughts away from your self and out into the world around you, your whole experience of that world can change and the answers that you are searching for will come to you.

Turning my attention away from myself gave me the most fascinating insight into the individuality of other people, and I learned to become much more flexible in my own behaviour. I learned that people need to be motivated in different ways. Some people need an approach that is very caring, while others need to be pushed. Others just want an outlet for their stress, to have fun, somebody to talk to. I had to draw on my own internal resources to get results out of people, and it was wonderfully rewarding to help my clients achieve their goals. I went from strength to strength in other areas of fitness and particularly enjoyed teaching ante- and post-natal exercise and children's fitness. I went on to write a regular column for a popular health magazine and present a number of videos. (So my time as a presenter had not been wasted.) I was still on occasion worried and anxious, and that caustic inner voice frequently made itself heard. But somehow I began to feel less burdened. Being active seemed to have triggered a sense that anything was possible if I really wanted it.

It is now well documented that physical fitness benefits you mentally. Exercise can bring about improvements in self-esteem and self-image and increase confidence. When our confidence and esteem are lifted our perception of ourselves changes completely. Exercise also releases hormones that affect your mood, creating a more relaxed and positive frame of mind and releasing physical stress from the body.

Exercise can bring about improvements in self-esteem, self-image and confidence.

Exercise also gives you time out by distracting you from your everyday problems. As you become physically stronger you become mentally stronger too. The brain works more efficiently and your ability to plan and organize, to focus, concentrate and be creative improves.

Physical fitness was a remarkably effective tool in leading me away from the state I was in. It was the first step for me on the way to achieving a balanced mind and body. But while I had become much more flexible in my approach to life, the internal saboteur still raged within; and while I had tried many different therapies in the past I still hadn't addressed my underlying feelings about myself. Because I now had two outlets – motherhood and work – I literally threw myself into them and tried to avoid the negative feelings that seemed to pop up so frequently. In retrospect I worked far too hard. I was teaching too much. My excuse was that the money that fitness professionals earned was so poor that I had to take the number of classes I did in order to make ends meet. In truth I was becoming unbalanced and the result was burn-out. I was now underweight, which in fact is just as problematic as being overweight. My own fitness levels had dropped and I was beginning to feel unfulfilled.

The human body is like a natural barometer, it tells you when something is not right, mentally and physically. We ignore our bodies' messages at our peril. Feelings do not disappear if we ignore them, they may fade for a little while but unless they are addressed they are likely to come back again and again. And the more we try to avoid the feedback from those messages the more insistent they can become. When your body tells you that you are imbalanced, you need to do something to move towards a state of balance. You can do this by changing your behaviour and your thinking. How we manage ourselves, how we act, the way we carry ourselves, the words we speak – all determine how well our lives work for us. When our actions are guided by positive messages things go much better for us.

The first step towards changing a negative state is awareness.

Moving On

After nearly ten years of living and breathing fitness I was restless, unfulfilled and tired. I became acutely aware of how my state of mind affected my exercise regime. I also became aware that some of my clients were making fantastic gains through their training while others seemed to make very little improvement. Often when we went jogging together they would open their hearts and tell me about their problems. I began to recognize patterns of behaviour that would cause their weight to fluctuate. It seemed that the happier they were, the easier the sessions would be; and the unhappier they were, the more I needed to motivate them. My mother used to tell me that I was like an old mother hen always clucking around people who needed help. But I was beginning to look like a very scrawny old hen. How could I help others without first helping myself? I began to give my thoughts and feelings some attention and was amazed at what I discovered about my own feelings towards exercise.

Although I have always had strong beliefs about how important it is to exercise, I couldn't always balance my behaviour with my reasoning mind. It seemed as if I was caught between two extremes. If I was having a good day I would be motivated to exercise and feel positive about life. But if I was having a challenging day I often had to really motivate myself to go to the gym. Just the sight of all that machinery made me feel that the next hour would be a real effort. I also found that I avoided many exercise classes because I used to worry about the footwork. I would respond well to anything sporty – such as circuit training – but often those classes did not fit with my busy schedule.

The turning point came when I went on a run by the Thames. It was a beautiful evening, and as I started off I was positively relishing the thought of a jog by the calm waters – but then the negative voice demanded to be heard. 'You will look such an idiot going past that pub with all those blokes watching you.' 'How much farther have I got to go?' 'Gosh, I'm so sweaty; it feels awful.' As my attention was on these restrictive thoughts a big Alsatian suddenly appeared in my path. I panicked. And that was it – I turned and ran all the way home.

At the time I laughed at the absurdity of my behaviour. However, it also gave me food for thought. I was becoming ever more aware of my state of mind and the effects of the negative self-talk. And its influence over my own exercise regime and my life generally.

Your 'state' is the sum total of your physiology, your thoughts and your emotions. It can change from moment to moment and can be either positive or negative. We give different states of mind labels like 'irritation', 'serenity', 'agitation'. Your state of mind affects the way that you think and your physiology, which then has an effect on the actions that you take. The first step towards changing a negative state is awareness. When we are more aware we become sensitive to the messages that come to us from the world around us and from within. The most underused but powerful of our natural resources, awareness brings these messages to full consciousness, which helps us to recognize how we may be restricting our responses on both the physical and mental levels. When we pay attention to the messages from within and without, we can then act to change those responses.

Tools for Change

Over the years I have tried all kinds of therapies to beat depression. I was and I still am always curious to try anything new. I had tried conventional therapies such as counselling and psychotherapy, but I found that I was naturally drawn to the more 'alternative' therapies such as reflexology, kineseology and spiritual healing. Of all the therapies I have experienced, the most effective was hypnotherapy, which enabled me to go from smoking 20 a day to being a non-smoker overnight. It also helped to build my confidence generally. But what we must realize is that hypnosis is simply a label for a state of mind that we all achieve every day of our

Your state of mind affects the way that you think and your physiology.

lives – when we daydream, for example, or in the moments before going off to sleep at night or when we awake in the morning. Other labels for this state might be called 'meditation', 'daydreaming', 'relaxation', 'trance', the 'reverie state', to name but a few. The amazing thing is that we can achieve this state whenever we want to and then guide our minds through suggestion and visualization. This can be incredibly useful in all areas of personal development. You simply have to learn to relax.

You probably think you already know how to relax. But it's not just about taking a rest or having a cup of tea or slumping in front of the telly. Your body and mind are capable of achieving a deep state of relaxation with untold benefits for both. Absolutely everyone can achieve this state when both body and mind are in complete harmony. When your body achieves balance and your mind is clear, the door to your inner world can be opened, and this allows you to take control of your own thought processes and develop your self-knowledge.

NLP

The other discipline that attracted me was Neuro-Linguistic Programming or NLP. I would describe NLP as a new way of thinking, an alternative form of psychology. NLP takes a very resourceful approach to life. It was originated in the 1970s in America by Richard Bandler and John Grinder, who were then respectively a student in psychology and mathematics and an assistant professor of linguistics. They believed that through curiosity and exploration you could 'model' excellence in all areas of life and explore your programming and experience. NLP focuses on what can be done to make fast, effective changes to people's lives by tapping into an individual's internal resources, creating positive behaviour patterns for the future. It examines how the different ways that people think and communicate with each other affect their lives. Using this method of thinking you can dramatically improve your attitude, your relationships and your performance in every area of your life.

A New Attitude

It was time to hang up my leotard and move on. I had finally found the means to sort out my life. I felt as though a magic wand had been waved and that I had been given the tools for a happy life. My outlook changed completely. I realized that as a result of the way I interpreted my experiences my map of the world was hugely distorted and did not in fact reflect my true abilities and potential. My entire life had been guided by this map of the world that I had created even though it was a map that was always getting me lost. As all of this finally sank in I began to draw up a new map underwritten by a more optimistic attitude, and positive beliefs and expectations. It was the most liberating feeling you can possibly imagine. My thinking about exercise began to change and that spiteful voice that had seemed in the past to constantly nag at me became

Choose to change today. It's time to get fit from the inside out as well as the outside in.

less harsh. My runs along the river became much more enjoyable. No dog would send me scurrying for home again. I ran in true Rocky style, ready to take on the world. Whenever I attended an exercise class it no longer mattered that I shot off in the opposite direction to everyone else. It simply didn't matter. And as I learned to control my own inner critic I realized that through my training in NLP and other therapies that I was now ready to really help others. I had truly awakened.

Take a good look at your own map of the world and ask yourself if you want this map to be true for you and if it is the one you want to live by. If you don't want it, you can change it. Because what you believe to be true and real determines your attitude toward life and affects all that you do. What this book will show you is how to develop your own experiences in ways that are more helpful to you. It will show you how to create a new map of the world by simply making the decision to change your thinking. Your whole attitude can alter if you want it to, and you can realize your dreams in every area of your life.

I believe that I discovered something that made all the difference to my attitude towards exercise. In fact, towards life. And if I did it, so can you. Each and every one of you has the most incredible resources that will enable you to achieve your exercise goals and to make changes in your life. All you need is the will and the desire to make those changes, to open your mind and then simply to put to good use the tools in this book. Choose to change today. It's time to get fit from the inside out as well as outside in.

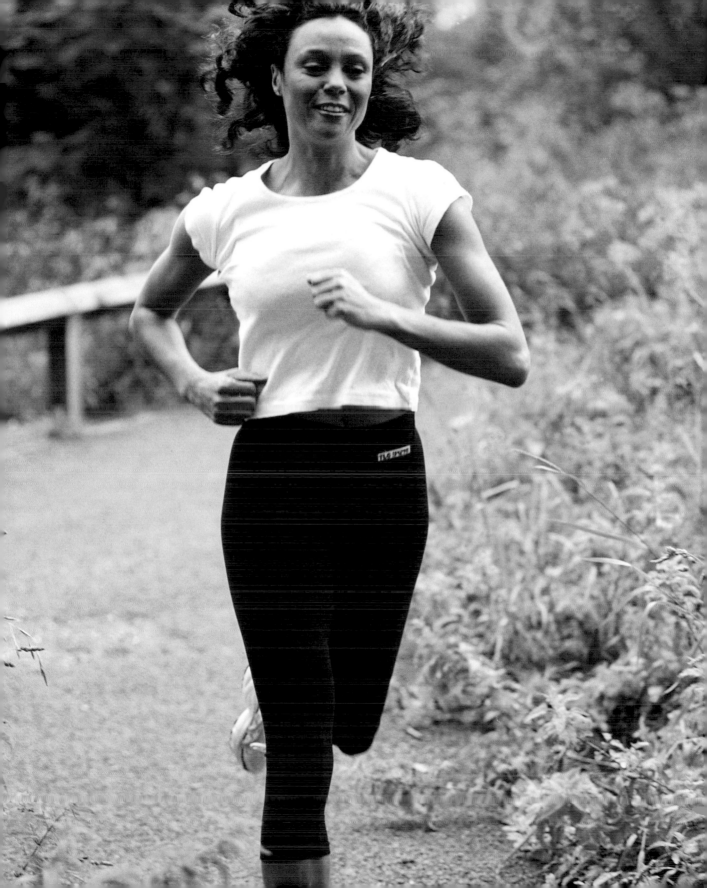

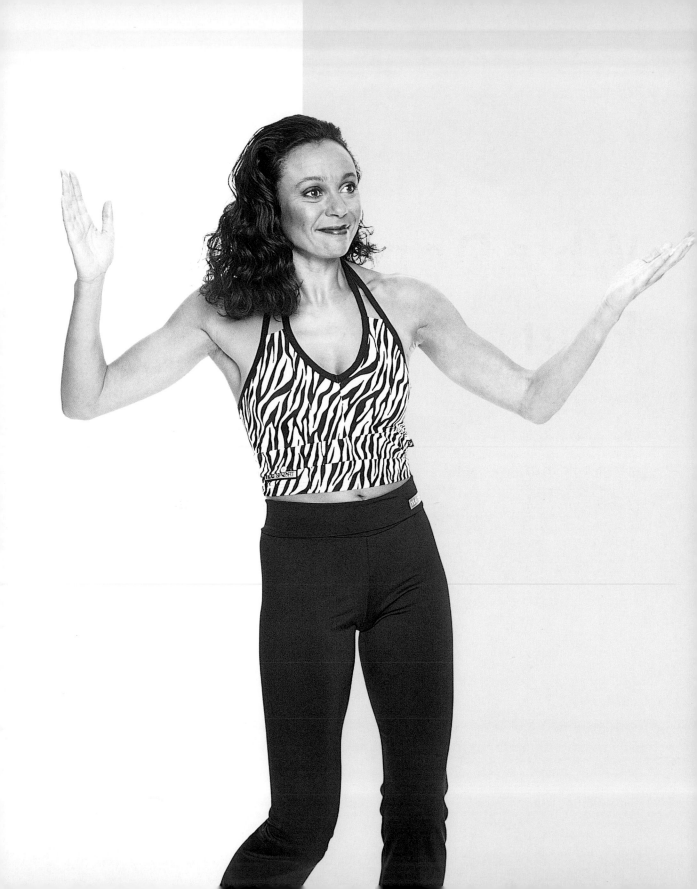

Chapter 2

Why Don't People Exercise?

Do you want to exercise but never really seem to? Is it too much of a chore for you and do fitness regimes soon get put aside? Do you have a negative attitude towards fitness in general? If any of these strikes a chord, don't worry – it seems that two-thirds of the adult population is with you.

Why Don't People Exercise?

A British Heart Foundation (BHF) survey found that only 37 per cent of men and 25 per cent of women are moderately active for the suggested 30 minutes five times a week. Furthermore, a 1997 Health Education Authority (HEA) survey and an Allied Dunbar survey of 1992 show that not only is a high percentage of the population not exercising but that the percentages change with age and gender. For example, between the ages of 16 and 24 women are less active than men: the HEA survey entitled 'What You Think' suggested that only 30 per cent of women, compared to 58 per cent of men, exercise for five 30-minute sessions a week. It also appears that women of this age group are less active then women who are 10 or 20 years older.

At the other end of the scale, around 40 per cent of all men and women aged 50 and over are sedentary, not managing even one 30-minute session in a week. Only one in four men and one in six women are frequently active beyond the age of 50. Another survey carried out by the BHF showed that only 17 per cent of men and 12 per cent of women aged 65 to 74 were active. Research was undertaken to see if people in this age group could walk a quarter of a mile without stopping or suffering discomfort. Only a quarter of the women and one-third of the men were able to do so!

And it is not only adults who are not using their bodies. With comfort and convenience being the norm, and cars, computers and television promoting inactivity, it is no surprise that our children are couch potatoes. One of the alarming findings of the BHF was that in England only 55 per cent of boys and 39 per cent of girls between the ages of 2 and 15 are moderately active for the recommended one hour a day.

These figures reveal a population disinclined towards fitness between the ages of 16 to 75. And yet why should this be the case? We all know the benefits of being fit. In the short term they are a better body shape, stronger, toned muscles, improved posture, a more positive outlook and more energy. In the long term physical activity promotes good health, prevents disease and has an important role to play in how we function on

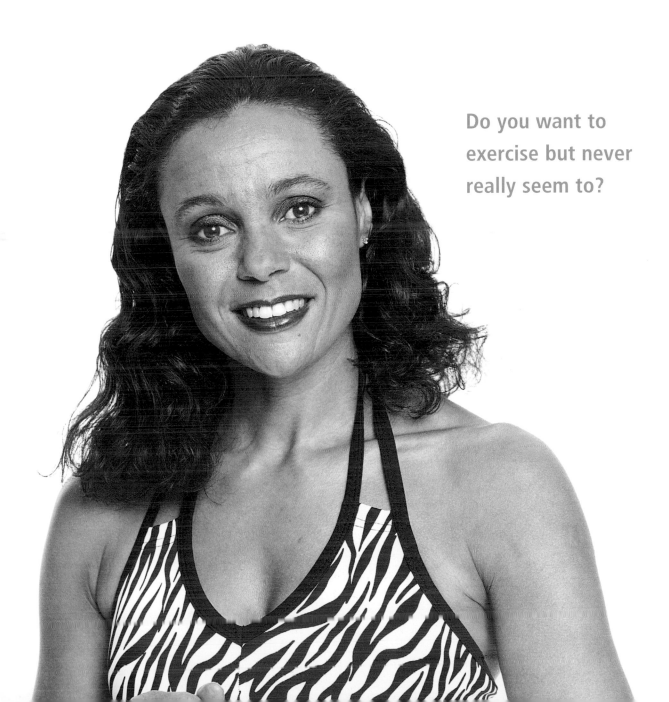

Do you want to
exercise but never
really seem to?

a day to day basis. So again, why, knowing all of this, don't we exercise enough? Allied Dunbar's national survey of 1992 suggests that a number of factors prevent people from making fitness a priority in their lives.

Factors that kept 16 to 69 year olds from activity

	Men%	Women%
I need to rest and relax in my spare time	25	26
I haven't got the energy	13	21
I'd never keep it up	12	19
I don't enjoy physical activity	9	13
I haven't got the time	41	43
I don't have time because of work	34	21
I've got young children to look after	10	18
There is no one to do it with	14	22
I can't afford it	9	14
I haven't got the right clothes	5	7
There are no facilities nearby	8	12
I am not the sporty type	24	38
I am too shy and embarrassed	4	12
I might get injured and damage my health	7	5
I have an injury or disability that stops me	18	15
I am too fat	7	14
My health is not good enough	11	7
I am too old	7	7

Many of the 16 to 24 year olds questioned for the HEA's ' What You Think' survey had their own reasons for not exercising, such as going to university and the need to earn a living. While the HEA's 'Later in Life' survey revealed that many older men and women think exercise is something best avoided on health grounds ('It might not be good for me'). Unfortunately, over 65 per cent of women over the age of 70 are completely sedentary and don't even have the strength to push themselves out of a chair. What is clear is that a lot of our time and most of our energy are taken up by things that we prioritize above exercise.

It is now time for you to explore what you think about exercise. I have divided what, in my experience, are the main reasons given for not exercising into three categories – physical, mental and emotional. Tick those that apply to you.

It is now time for you to explore what you think about exercise.

Physical

- I am too fat
- I have an injury that stops me
- It is too much physical effort
- I never know if I am doing the exercise correctly
- There are no facilities close enough
- I give up if I don't see immediate results
- My body is not made for exercise
- Exercise hurts
- I physically can't keep up so I give up

Emotional

- I don't have the confidence to get started
- I start full of enthusiasm and then give up after a few weeks
- I'm just not good at it
- My moods affect whether I do it or not
- I feel inadequate because I never seem to reach my goals
- I do not enjoy exercise
- I am terribly self-conscious in all health clubs
- I hate the way I look in exercise gear
- I am easily inhibited by others in classes

Mental

- I don't believe that I can reach my goals
- I can't be bothered
- I cannot find a form of exercise to suit me
- The weather puts me off
- I exercise half-heartedly
- I don't know how to
- It's simply too big a task
- I haven't got the time
- I have no one to exercise with

There are no right or wrong answers here and no adding up marks to label yourself 'good', 'bad' or 'indifferent'. Clearly, the more ticks you made the more resistance you may feel towards exercise. The fewer ticks you made the fewer issues you have with exercise and the more positive your outlook will be.

Take a look again at the ticks that you made. Is there any one group that has more ticks than others? If the ticks are evenly spread, is there a particular area that you want to work on? If there is, write it down now.

*Imagine
that there is a six-inch-wide plank of wood
lying on the floor. Now imagine yourself walking across
that plank. It's so easy isn't it? Now I'd like you to imagine that
you are at the top of a ten-story building with the same plank
stretched between two buildings. Now try to walk across it.
You will probably find that you will have great
difficulty in doing so.*

The Essential Ingredient

Whether your reasons for not exercising are physical, mental or emotional, or a combination of these, you will find that there is one essential factor that underlies them all: your will and your desire to get fit. Often you may think that you can will yourself to do anything, that you can get by on will-power alone. But the old saying – 'where there's a will there's a way' – is not always true. When you will yourself – no matter how hard – to do something that you really don't desire to do, you may well find that your efforts end in failure. Your will-power comes from the conscious mind, which is the reasoning part of your mind. Your desire comes from the subconscious mind which houses your imagination, memories, motivation and energy. Whenever there is a battle between reason and your emotions, your emotions will win.

When I did the exercise above I wobbled a lot and then fell off. What happened? My imagination was more powerful than my will. As much as I tried to will myself to walk across the plank, I believed that I would fall even though I tried not to. Reason told me that I was on an imaginary plank of wood on my living room floor but my imagination insisted that I was ten floors above ground – and I felt all the uncertainty I would have if I really had been attempting that feat. If you don't really desire to exercise – and imagine you will fail or feel that it is a chore – but you try and force yourself to do it, it is unlikely you will enjoy exercise or exercise for long – if at all.

Think about a time when you really desired to do something. What happened? Did all of you desire this or only part of you? Did you follow through this desire? Try to recapture that experience as fully as you can. What do you see? What are you saying to yourself. How do you feel?

Now think about exercise. Think about a past experience of physical activity. What is the degree of your desire now? What do you see? What are you saying to yourself? How do you feel?

Exercise Drop-out

You may desire to get fit and start full of good intentions but somehow you seem to slack off and lose interest. The message that you may be telling yourself is that the effort is too much, or that there is something more important you should be dealing with. You may find that you lost the desire to exercise in the time it took you to get to the gym. Or perhaps other things that are more important to you get in the way. You find that the intensity of your initial desire diminishes and you talk yourself out of getting fit.

If, on thinking back to an experience of exercise, your level of desire is lower, explore the reasons why. How is the remembered exercise different from the first experience? How are they similar? How could you increase your desire to exercise? How does the language you used to describe the two experiences differ. If your language was negative or maybe just non-committal when it came to exercise, try to think why. Now think how you could increase your desire to exercise to tip the balance.

Ultimately the million-dollar question is: Do you *want* to have the will and desire to exercise assuming you could find a way to do it? Yes, no or don't know?

If you thought 'no' and don't think that you even want to have the will then we're in trouble: nobody can make you want what you don't desire. In fact, we very rarely do what we least want to do. So if you really don't want to put one foot in front of the other and get fit you won't. If you mentally ticked 'don't know' then that's a start, because it means that you are ready to explore a little further (and let's face it, you didn't buy this book in order to give up at chapter 2). Keep reading. If you mentally ticked 'yes' then the next step for you is to make a committed decision to keep fit and then to find the stimulus to keep you going until you reach your goals.

You get what you focus on.

Decisions

We make decisions every day of our lives, some big and some small. Sometimes we are indecisive and cannot make up our minds about something until we have processed enough information to reach a conclusion. Sometimes we change the decisions we make if the consequences don't quite suit us. When it comes to exercise, people can make a decision to get fit or lose weight and then quickly unmake it, as the desire is dissipated by the effort it takes and the hurdles life puts in the way.

In order to make a decision about something you have to focus your attention on it. If you focus on something that you really like then you are likely – surprise, surprise – to make a decision to move towards it. And vice versa. What you focus on – and its desirability or otherwise – affects the way that you feel and influences the decisions you make.

Pain and Pleasure

Pain and pleasure influence the decisions we make. Pleasure we are drawn to, pain we try to avoid. Anything in between the two we tolerate. Pain can manifest itself physically or emotionally (as fear, anxiety, even lethargy and boredom). Although pain is uncomfortable, it is essential. It tells us to pay attention to what we are doing and to take action. But we have a tendency to react instantaneously to an uncomfortable feeling rather than give it any attention. There are times when what we really need to do is to look beyond our immediate discomfort and make a considered decision rather than reacting thoughtlessly.

Imagine you are meeting a friend, someone with whom you can easily speak your mind. Imagine that he or she asks how you really feel about exercising. Jot down quickly your spontaneous – and therefore honest – answer. Now look at what you wrote. It is likely to reflect your internal dialogue about and during actual exercise.

Now read out loud what you wrote down. Listen to your tone of voice. Ask yourself: If I were a personal trainer would I choose those words and that tone to motivate others? If your words are negative then try it again with the following in mind: choose a friendly tone of voice; make positive suggestions such as 'You can ...'; keep focusing on the benefits of exercise.

Exercise

Often exercise is perceived to be an uncomfortable experience. You may find that when you start to exercise you can experience a challenge to your body and your mind. Your mind and body give you feedback – and the inevitable internal dialogue can start up, often distorting your experience. I remember a client I took out for a gentle run. Within minutes he was pulling faces. He had made the decision in his mind that it was going to hurt and he made the run tough for himself in his head. He told everybody that I was a stern taskmaster but in fact he wasn't even out of breath. He even managed to have a conversation with me. He was simply distorting the experience in his mind. When I made him aware of this he was able to relax and enjoy himself much more next time around.

Internal Dialogue

Often when we encounter fitness challenges we decide 'I am so unfit' or 'I will never be able to keep this up.' Or if we don't see the results immediately we decide that it is not worth the effort. But in reality the opposite is true. Every time we exercise we are doing our body some good. Every time we take action we are working towards improving or at least maintaining our fitness levels. Every time you exercise you can congratulate yourself on a small victory. But if during exercise you focus on how awful

Look back at the survey of reasons for not exercising. Do you think that they are valid reasons? For example, the biggest problem seems to be time. Do we really not have time to exercise? Surely, if we desired it enough we would find the time. Think about the areas you yourself ticked. Looking back at it now, would you say that – apart from physical injury – there are any valid reasons for not exercising. Yes or no?

If 'yes', then do you think it is worth finding ways to work either through or around this reason so that you can find a way? If 'no', are you ready to make a commitment to the time it will take?

you feel or how unfit you are, the more you begin to believe it. And that's what makes you want to stop. So how do you cope with the discomfort that is integral to really beneficial exercise? By acknowledging those feelings of discomfort as momentary sensations and learning to tolerate them in the knowledge that they are making you fitter and healthier. See the discomfort for what it really is. Focus on the positive aspects of exercise and you will be amazed at how much you are able to tolerate and even enjoy. Paying attention to your feelings can transform your experience of them.

We all have a unique view of the world and our attitudes to life are all different. Some of us are naturally more optimistic about life and others more pessimistic. And this optimism or pessimism reveals itself in your physiology and in the language you use both internally and externally. If you have a positive attitude you are more likely to have an upright, 'lifted' posture and a smile on your face, to walk with a spring in your step and use positive language (remember 'You can ...'). Equally, we all recognize the outward manifestations of a negative attitude towards life ('I can't ...' or 'I'll never be able to').

Attitude – Positive and Negative

Your attitude reflects your mental and physical being. Where does this attitude come from? The answer is your conditioning and the language that you use: all that we have absorbed from family, friends, school and the world around us. What we learn from our life's experience is internalized, repeated and habituated and ultimately forms our attitude to life.

- Watch your thoughts: they become words
- Watch your words: they become actions
- Watch your actions: they become habits
- Watch your habits: they become your character
- Watch your character: it becomes your destiny

In today's society it is easy to focus on the negatives. Every day the papers, radio and television bring us heart-rending stories from around the world; every day heralds a new disaster. A report from a leading UK charity states that one in five people in the UK suffer from depression. It is thought that by 2020 depression will be the second most troublesome condition in the world. These figures are overwhelming, as is the sheer weight of the negative messages that surround us. If we absorb these messages we find that they can have an effect on our state of mind and on the decisions we make.

So your thoughts and the way you focus on them play a significant role in determining your attitude to life. If you think positively you are more likely to use positive language inside your head, which will colour the words that you hear outside your head. A positive attitude means positive decisions, which will help you achieve your dreams. Think about all the people you know who have a positive attitude. Are they healthy, happy, and successful in their own way? Where exercise and fitness are concerned, a positive attitude means that you are likely to make positive decisions about physical activity. It means that you will be more likely to use positive language to talk yourself into exercising consistently – and enjoying it. If you think negatively you are likely to be less healthy and make limiting decisions, which may stop you from reaching your potential in every area of your life. Think about all the pessimistic people you know. Are they healthy? Do they sell themselves short and fail to achieve their goals? A negative attitude towards exercise will soon find you all the excuses you need to prevent you from becoming fit.

What about you? What is your general attitude towards life? Do you tend to be more optimistic or pessimistic? Is the glass half full or half empty? (This may be something of a cliché, but it's a very revealing cliché.) And what is your attitude towards exercise? Do you look forward to it and focus on how fantastic you are going to feel and look – or do you just think how useless you are and what a chore it all is?

The language you use is determined by your attitude – and how you choose to explain things to yourself makes a huge difference to your success or failure in exercise. After all, it is the language you will use to talk yourself into or out of exercising.

Think
about your experience of exercise and how
you respond when you come up against some sort of
hurdle, i.e. a new skill to learn or a time constraint. Do you talk
yourself through the challenge and keep going no matter what,
or do you tell yourself that it's not worth it and talk yourself
out of doing it? What do you say to yourself?

Just
think about how a positive attitude towards
exercise would help you reach your goals, be they short term or
long term. Practise using positive language to talk yourself into
exercising, performing to or above your expectations, praising yourself when
you do well and encouraging yourself when you are challenged. Imagine
yourself as your own personal trainer. If you were your own personal trainer
how would you respond when you needed help and support to
maintain and increase your fitness levels. How would you
make exercise more pleasurable?

The purpose of the following questions is to increase your awareness of your own attitude – positive or negative – towards exercise and to explore the benefits that having a positive mental attitude towards fitness will bring you. Ask yourself the following questions. As you work through them analyze your attitude and ask yourself if you want to change.

- Do I want to start making positive decisions towards exercise?
- What do I need to do to start making positive decisions towards exercise?
- How much time and effort can I commit to putting this into practise?
- Who else would be involved?
- When will I do this?
- What is the next step from here?

Do I want to start making positive decisions towards exercise? Yes I do!

Congruent Behaviour

It's natural to have mixed feelings about many things in life, and exercise is certainly an area ripe for conflict. I'm sure you've all had that battle with yourself, the one that sees you make a conscious decision to go to the gym but somehow not get there – and end up doing something completely different. Ever made the decision to get up early in the morning to exercise and then when it comes to the alarm going off your head is saying 'Come on, get a move on: you have exercise to do', but your heart is saying, 'It's so warm and snug ... just five more minutes. Just five more minutes. Just five more minutes.' Yes, as we've seen, your heart will usually win. (And then you have to deal with the telling off you give yourself later.)

I have a wonderful friend called Jennifer who was incredibly health conscious and wanted to exercise regularly and consistently. But when she tried to do anything about it she would have these feelings of complete rebellion and find ways to sabotage her efforts. Normally with a cigarette and a glass of wine! After working on her behaviour I managed to reach an agreement with the rebellious part of her that exercise was worth it and that it would benefit her. Jennifer now trains in the park and does yoga every morning.

When you are 'congruent' body and mind are in complete harmony and agreement. (Jennifer became congruent when the self-saboteur acknowledged the benefits of exercise and joined forces with her health-conscious side.) It is a state of mind to which success in all areas of life is attributed. Successful athletes are congruent in their behaviour, so are successful business people. When you are congruent in your attitude towards exercise you are more likely to decide to find a way to get and stay fit.

Think of two occasions on which you have been congruent in your behaviour. (The signs are positive body language backed up by positive language; an upbeat tone of voice; a passion for, about or to do something.) How did you feel physically? What do you remember seeing and hearing? Can you recapture your inner dialogue? What actions did you take as a result of being congruent?

Now think of two occasions on which you have been incongruent. (Characterized by the mixed message – you saying one thing and your body language another – or a sense of being pulled in different directions.) Do you remember how you felt and what you saw and heard? How did the inner dialogue run? What actions did you – or didn't you – take as a result of being incongruent?

Are you congruent in your thoughts about fitness? What lets you know that you are congruent? How do you feel physically? What is your thinking? What decisions do you make and do you put them into practice? Are they consistent? Are you congruent all of the time or only part of the time?

Imagine any of the conflicting parts of yourself as actors on a stage below and in front of you. Give them names. Establish gender. Pay attention to each part and find out about them. Ask each one to reveal their highest intention, that which is most important for them to achieve. Have them go on until they discover what they ultimately want (it is often the same thing) – it could be happiness, joy, freedom or safety. Then ask these actors to come up with ideas for working together to reach their shared goal more easily.

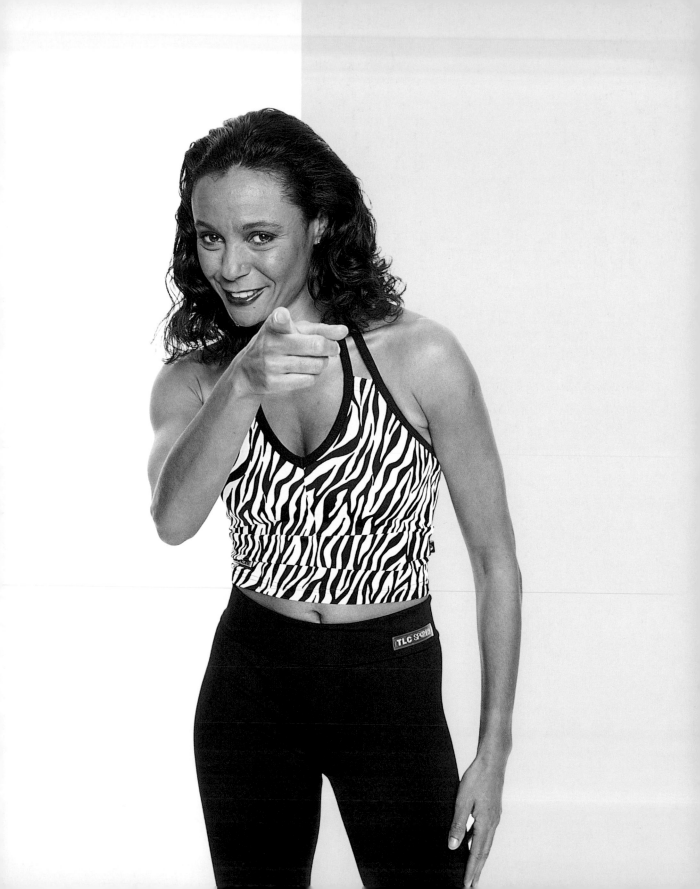

Chapter 3

Motivation

Motivation is that which has the power to cause you to act. It is motivation that gets you out of bed to exercise. It is motivation that makes you grit your teeth to do those extra sit-ups, and it is motivation that enables you to put your heart and soul into your workout.

Motivation

There are two types of motivation: positive and negative. At first the only kind of motivation we know is positive: think about young children and the way they always move towards what they want in an optimistic way. When we are motivated towards something it is generally something that we really want, like and value, something that gives us pleasure and in which we are prepared to invest time, energy and effort. Positive motivation is a feeling of being pulled towards something. It is the combination of will-power and desire and it is the most important ingredient in achieving success.

Think of a time when you experienced negative motivation. Perhaps something you had to do but didn't want to. As you recall what you were moving away from, recapture what you saw, heard and felt at the time.

As life and the world around us condition us we learn negative motivation. When you are motivated away from something you feel as though you are acting against your will. So if you are negatively motivated to exercise you are likely to do it because you want to avoid something else, such as a heart attack or becoming overweight. When a person experiences negative motivation, often they talk about what they don't want and tend to focus on problems that may arise.

Exercise is an area where the different types of motivation stand out. There is positive and negative motivation (and of course there is no motivation at all to exercise. Which means that you are simply not interested – and no one can force you to become motivated.) One way of identifying the nature of your motivation is to listen carefully to the language that you use both internally and externally. Whenever you say 'Oh no, I should go to the gym' or 'I really need to lose weight' you are manifesting negative motivation. Whenever you say 'I want to exercise' or 'I am off to the gym' you are positively motivated. What are your feelings towards exercise? Are you motivated towards it or away from the dangers of not exercising?

We all have different reasons to be motivated to exercise. We can be motivated out of necessity. As time goes by and we become more inactive

*Think
of something that you have really
wanted and went all out to get. Recall what
you were doing, what you saw, heard and felt at
the time. Relive the situation and the
feelings as fully as you can.*

the inevitable happens: our metabolism slows down, we begin to lose our muscle mass and our body fat increases. Poor postural habits begin to kick in and you can be left feeling plain unhealthy. If you exercise out of necessity then you are likely to say to yourself 'I have to do it', 'I really should go to the gym today.' We can also be motivated out of a sense of possibility, of the opportunities that may arise from a new situation. Exercise raises the possibility of a new body shape or fitness challenge or even of meeting a new partner.

If you are positively motivated to exercise you are more likely make sure that you do it, to imagine your fitness goals for the future and to be prepared to work through the process that will achieve them. If you are negatively motivated to exercise you will probably still go through with it, but you are likely to think that fitness is a chore and to focus on the problems involved in getting fit, and you are likely to focus on the short-term benefits rather than the long-term achievements.

However, you can change your motivation from negative to positive by changing your perception and making fitness a more pleasurable experience. If you can make it more fun and find ways and means of working through your resistance, you can actually look forward to going through the process of exercise and reaping the benefits of a strong, fit body.

Your Feelings

Negative feelings can influence your decision to exercise. The Allied Dunbar survey revealed that the second commonest resistance to exercise came from our emotions. Twenty-four per cent of men and 38 per cent of women allow limiting beliefs and other negative emotional states of mind to prevent them exercising. The main problem is the notion that you need to be sporty to do exercise. And if you are feeling pessimistic, down, depressed or prone to mood swings you are more likely to talk yourself out of than into exercise. Often the thought of physical activity can trigger memories of perceived failures on the school field and in competition with others, of feelings of self-consciousness and 'exposure' and of low self-esteem caused by negative body image. These feelings can be painful and we naturally seek to avoid their cause. These experiences create feelings that can become habitual and ingrained in some of us, and they will always limit us unless we do something to change them. Here are a number of typical sentiments I have encountered.

- 'I couldn't go to the gym. It's far too intimidating.'
  (21 year old)
- 'I've got stretch marks, I have to run from the changing room to the pool.' (18 year old)
- 'I just can't do it.' (51 year old)
- 'I drive to the gym and then I sit outside. I don't have the confidence to go in.'(35 year old)
- 'You have to be thin to go to a health club.'
  (43 year old)

These feelings of vulnerability are more likely to be provoked by past experiences and negative feedback that are now habitually associated with exercise. Once these statements are ingrained we can become stuck with them and feel powerless to move on – because we do not know that we can choose to do so.

Below is a list of feelings that are commonly associated with exercise. Are any of these feelings familiar to you? Is there one feeling that you know better than the others? Have any of these feelings become habitual to you?

positive

- Confidence
- Excitement
- Relaxed
- Focus
- Determination
- Empowerment
- Motivation
- Purposefulness

negative

- Fear
- Self-consciousness
- Boredom
- Worry
- Frustration
- Tension
- Depression
- Anxiety

If you had both positve and negative responses what is the difference between the two sets of feelings? Which feeling would you prefer to have? Hopefully you will see how easy it is to access different feelings and how we can create positive feelings if we choose to.

Sit in a relaxed and comfortable position and pick a negative label from the list. Close your eyes and recall an experience of this feeling. As you relive the experience just be aware of how quickly the feeling comes to you. Then come back to the present and change your state by standing up or walking around.

Now choose a positive label. Recall an experience of this feeling. Again, be aware of how quickly this feeling comes to you. Now just allow the feeling to grow and grow inside you. When the feeling is at its peak, think of a word or a picture that will allow you to trigger this feeling at will.

Taking time out to exercise helps to put things into perspective.

Taking Control

We can control our emotions if we choose to, and we can change negative emotions to positive ones. How? Firstly, by making the choice to take control of our emotions instead of allowing them to control us. Secondly, by discovering and utilizing the resources that enable us to create change both internally and externally. One of the presuppositions of NLP is that we have the resources within us to excel in every area of our lives. We just need to access those resources and find ways to put them to good use! And it's worth repeating: we have the resources within us to excel in every area of our lives.

Just knowing this makes us realize that there is so much (more) we can do and achieve. In the past we have placed too much emphasis on the doing and not on the processing that happens in our minds beforehand. What makes us successful in life is the way we process information (in its widest sense). What is so interesting is that in this country we have been reluctant to address the 'how-tos' at a mental and emotional level. We have placed all our emphasis on the 'how-tos' at a physical level. But if you address your state of mind, you actually find that you have the motivational tools that will allow you to work through your resistance to fitness. These are tools that will help you to take control and train your mind to get you to where you want to be – in fitness and in life. It's time now to train your mind from the inside out to empower you to achieve your exercise goals.

To change a negative emotional state it helps to know where it originates. The exercise on the opposite page will show you how to do just that.

Sit or lie in a comfortable position. Close your eyes and relax. As you focus on your breathing allow your body to relax a little more. Now pay attention to a negative feeling that that is familiar to you. Be aware of where you feel it in your body. (Usually we 'feel' in the solar plexus area or the stomach.) Ask this feeling where it comes from and explore its origins. Ask this feeling what its purpose is for you. How is this purpose useful? Listen for its answer. Thank the feeling for its response and if it has anything to tell you. As you listen to the response, are you aware of having learned something that may allow you to let go of the negative emotion?

Imagine a part of you that is wiser than this 'feeling' part. Allow it to go to this feeling part and fill it with words of wisdom. This will bring about a new awareness that will allow you to let go of the negative emotion. Look inside yourself again. Where and what are the emotions now?

Apply this exercise to other events in your life that have triggered negative feelings and let them all go. Work through as many as you can. Allow the process – achieving awareness of the source of negative feeling and substituting positives – to take place in your mind and body. Now test the future. Imagine an event in the future that in the past would have set off negative feelings. Can you see a different result?

Creating Space

Our great plans for exercise sometimes just seem to fall through. Often this is because negative emotions stifle our motivation. We waste a lot of time dwelling on the stresses of life. Taking time out to exercise is actually the answer to this. Exercise distracts the mind, freeing it up and allowing us to be creative. Exercise can be good therapy. The purpose of the next exercise is to create space in the mind. To change a negative feeling we need to change our thinking or change our physiology – the way we hold ourselves affects our state of mind.

*Sit
and relax and turn your attention to how you
are feeling. Are you happy, sad, relaxed, agitated or ...? Are
these feelings coming from part of you or all of you? Is there a particular
issue on your mind? Does this issue relate to past, present or future? Imagine
that you are writing these thoughts down on a piece of paper. When you have
written them down see yourself folding up the paper and putting it away. Now be
aware of your mind becoming clear. Listen to your inner personal trainer
encouraging you to take time out for a walk, a yoga session, an aerobics
class. Make an agreement with yourself that while your worry is
put away your creative mind will work on a
permanent solution.*

*Think
of a time when you were down and
depressed. As you recall that time allow your body
to reflect your feelings at the time. Your shoulders are
rounded and pushed forward. You are breathing high in
your chest. Your head is hanging down
and your facial expression is
suitably downcast.*

*Take
a moment to shake off those negative
feelings. Now think of an incident when you were
really positive and motivated. As you recall the
experience allow the positive feeling to flood into your
body. Be aware of the changes that are taking place.
Your shoulders are upright, your head held high
and your body is lifted. Now smile.*

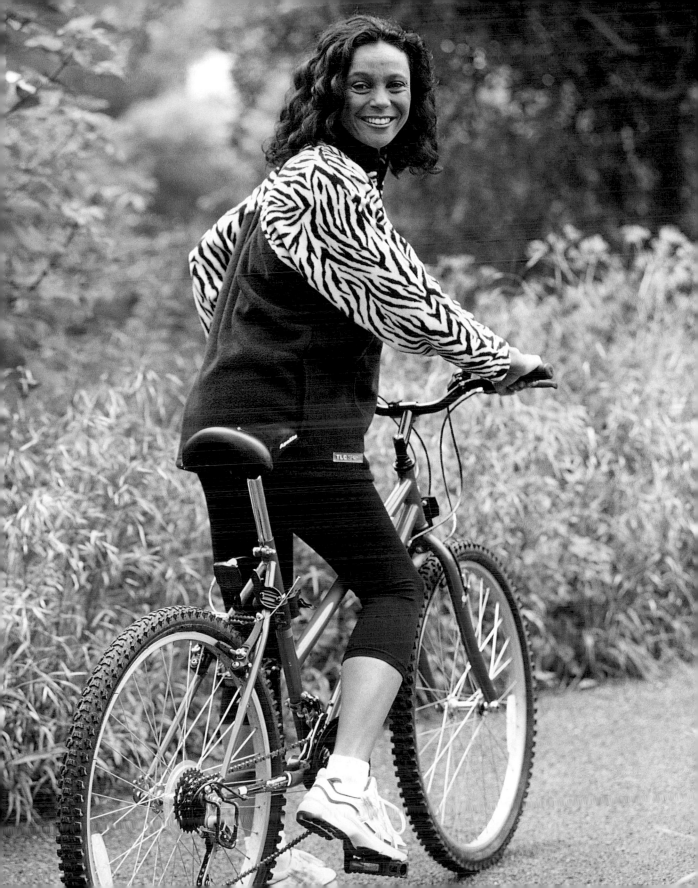

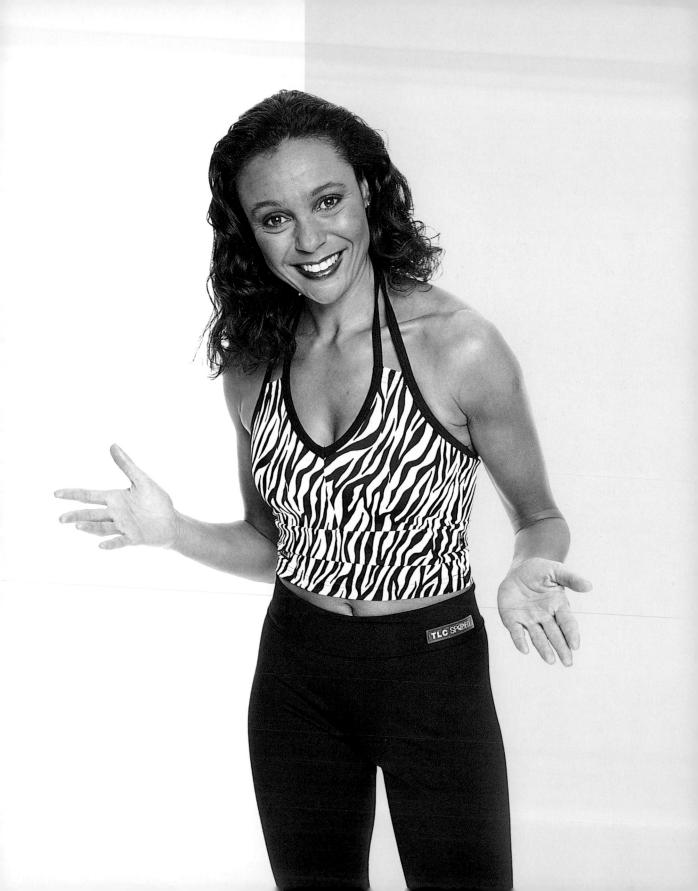

Environment

We take in information from the outside world through our senses. This information has an effect on our internal environment, influencing our thoughts and feelings and state of mind, which in turn has an effect on the decisions we make and our behaviour. Now, for our purposes, the 'environment' is that outside world: everything around you that can affect your state of mind and the choices that you make. The colour of the sky, the air that you breathe, the flowing water of a river, the autumn leaves, the sounds that you hear around you, the people you interact with, the quality of the food that you eat, the place in which you work – everything is significant.

Now put pen to paper and jot down some notes of your impressions of your environment. Is your environment pleasing to your senses, are you aware of something you might not normally pay attention to?

Take a moment to relax. Take a few deep breaths. Now take your awareness outside yourself to the environment around you. What do you see? Are you indoors or outdoors? Look at the space around you, what colours do you see? As you look and pay attention to what you see you may become aware of having to take in a lot of information. You may ordinarily delete what you do not need to see and focus on only what is useful and pleasurable. But just take a moment to do the opposite. *See what you see*. Now take your awareness to the sounds around you. There may be silence, perhaps music, perhaps aeroplanes flying overhead or the sound of the washing machine. *Hear what you hear*. As you pay attention to all that you experience around you, become aware of how the environment makes you feel. Do you have a sense of space, of calm and relaxation or are you surrounded by people and noise? *Feel what you feel*.

For example: 'As I look around me I see a cluttered room full of papers. I feel a great sense of space as I look through the French doors and see the rain pouring down. The colours in the room are quite relaxing

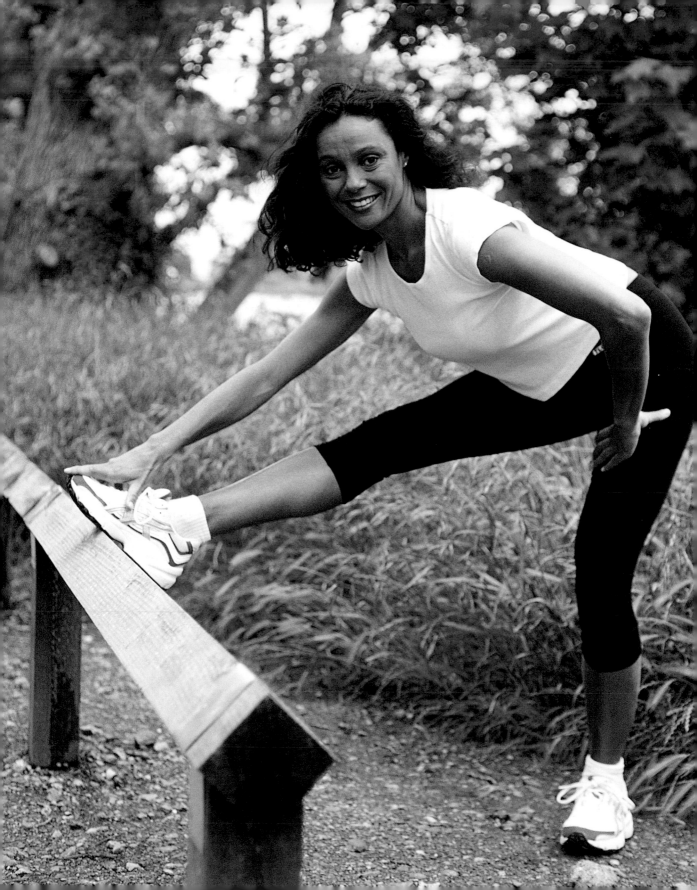

Your environment heavily influences the decisions that you make.

despite the clutter. I hear the sound of traffic in the distance, of someone mowing their lawn and my relaxation CD playing gently in the background.' How was it for you?

Your environment heavily influences the decisions that you make. As far as exercise is concerned, some people are put off because of the environment they are in or think that they have to be in. I have just stopped my membership at a health club where the environment was squeaky clean and perfect but lacked character. I need to feel that my exercise environment has been lived in. Also, there was no one to talk to, and if you can't have a chat with people while you work out, well, for me it's time to move on.

Some people won't set foot inside a gym because they are intimidated by machines. I had a client once who had very little confidence. She would drive to her local health club and then proceed to sit outside it for the next hour. She just did not feel comfortable about entering an alien environment. Think about the pain and pleasure connection from the last chapter. We also defined pain as uncomfortable feedback – what feedback do you get from your environment?

I have a really positive sense of space and freedom that I associate with my school sports day; I can remember people cheering me on. But I can also remember being put off a little later on by dirty, smelly changing rooms, classes that were so full of people that you couldn't move and other people's sweat all over the mats. Not nice.

Now what about your present experience with exercise. If you are exercising at all, are you exercising inside or outside? If you are exercising

Find ten minutes today to clear your mind and take a moment to think about a past experience with sport or exercise. Was your environment pleasant? As you recall your experience, just imagine you are back there. See what you were seeing, hear what you were hearing and feel what you were feeling. Jot down some notes about your past experience.

outside, does the weather affect your consistency? It might be useful to have some strategies in place for weather conditions. If you are a member of a health club, what is the environment like? What are the staff like – do they make you want to come back or are they grumpy? Did they mindlessly put you through your fitness induction and leave you clueless as to what to do? Is social environment important to you? Are you relaxed and at ease and comfortable in your current exercise environment. If you are at home, what is it like exercising alone? Do you have enough space around you to leap around to a step or aerobics video? Do you have enough space to lie down and do your stretches? When do you exercise – morning, afternoon or evening? How does that affect your state of mind? Sometimes we can simply set ourselves up for failure by choosing the wrong time of day.

Jot down some thoughts about your present experience.

You may now have a clearer idea about what environment has worked for you and what hasn't. You should also be aware of how your present experience of your exercise environment is affecting your decisions.

Now just take your time and imagine the type of environment in which you would like to exercise in the future. Perhaps a noisy studio full of people rampaging around isn't for you. Perhaps the silence and warmth of a yoga studio is more to your taste. Maybe you want to change with the seasons – winter inside, summer outside. What time do you want to exercise? What about clothing – what are you comfortable in? If you are exercising at home, how will you prepare and set up your exercise space? Who else will be there? If you have a child who is going to distract you, you will never be in the right frame of mind to focus on your exercise regime. We all deserve time for ourselves even when we have small children. What about the time factor? Is there any point in joining a health club that is a 20-minute drive away if you are short on time? If time is the issue, how can you make good use of what time you do have to do your exercise? When my son was small I would exercise in his naptime. I would

Focus on the ideal exercise environment for you for the future.

do a yoga workout and create a relaxing environment by lighting some candles, turning the telephone off and putting on some gentle music. By the time my son woke up I was considerably less frazzled than when I started. It was worth putting the effort in for this alone.

So what happens if you don't have an ideal environment? Although environment plays a very important part in the decisions you make about exercise, it is too easy to use a less than perfect environment as an excuse not to exercise. No matter what your situation, you can build a positive exercise environment around you. You just have to create it and make it happen.

For example, as I write this book with a deadline to meet I am limited to doing the New York City Ballet Workout on video first thing in the morning or exercising with my dynaband at around 11 o'clock at night while I watch the telly. A couple of times a week I can go for a run by the river. This may not be ideal, but I'm happy that it is as much as I can do in my current situation.

Behaviour

Our behaviour is what we say and what we do, what we 'express' externally – even when we aren't aware of it – to the world around us. It is the actions we take as a result of the inner dialogue we have with ourselves and the way we have been conditioned to approach life. All behavioural patterns are learned, and our parents and those around us when we are growing up heavily influence our behaviour. So, if your parents were completely inactive, and unless they encouraged you to do otherwise, you may have 'learned' to be a couch potato too.

I remember being completely frustrated when I taught children's exercise classes. Sometimes I would have 25 in a class and then the next week only six. The classes were pure play and the children loved them (leaving the kids exhausted, much to the delight of their parents). But it

Take ten minutes today to relax, pen and paper in hand ready to make some notes about your behaviour. Are you consistent in the things that you do in life or are you erratic, tending to extremes? Are your actions in life generally positive or negative? What about your behaviour towards exercise? Listen to the language you use as you explore your behaviour. Is it positive or are you beating yourself up? The language that you use guides your behaviour. How is your internal language guiding you?

was the parents' behaviour that caused the fluctuations in attendance. Often the parents would drop the children off so that they could go shopping, but if they had something else to do or if it was raining they wouldn't show up (even though the classes were indoors). The parents did not take the exercise seriously enough, but it was the children who missed out. It was most interesting that the parents who were consistent in their own exercise regimes showed up, but many of those who weren't, didn't – and in turn passed down this attitude to their children. Look back to the statistics on children and activity in the first chapter and you can see the importance of learning consistent behavioural patterns when young.

In the past my own behaviour has been inconsistent. When I was up, I was up – positive and ready to take on the world. I would go for it in the gym or in my exercise programme. And when I was down I was sure to stay down. The negative self-talk would lead me round in circles and result in self-limiting decisions and negative actions. I would still pitch up for classes or a session in the gym, but somehow I found it difficult to put the same amount of effort in or I would work out half-heartedly.

Hopefully, you have become more aware of what it is you do. Have you been honest with yourself? It is important now that you don't make judgements about your behaviour, whether it is serving you well or not. There is no such thing as failure in these exercises, no right or wrong way to behave. I would suggest only that you have an awareness of the consequences of your behaviour and whether it is positive or negative and whether, ultimately, it is useful to you or not.

Habitual Behaviour

Every experience we have leaves its mark on the brain's 'receiving station': the cortex. The cortex is responsible for transforming information into action. The first time you perform an action, new neural connections are made in the brain. The more you repeat an action the easier it becomes to perform. So whatever we do, we can be said to be practising. But practice doesn't always make perfect – it is perhaps more accurate to say that practice makes permanent. Repeated actions become ingrained whether they are positive or negative – your brain doesn't differentiate. So if you repeat to yourself a statement such as 'I am hopeless at exercise', you will find that you will be hopeless or at best half-hearted. However, if you have really positive associations with exercise and think 'I'm really good at this' every time you repeat a particular thought, your experience will be positive and you're more likely to be successful. Every time you repeat a thought or a movement you get better and better at it – whether its effect is positive or negative, empowering or limiting.

I remember a habitual pattern of my own. I decided that I would confine my exercise to the studio where I could work out to music. I made a limiting decision that the gym was boring, and every time I walked through it to get to the studio I pulled a face at the machinery there. When I eventually got round to working out in the gym, the feelings triggered by the machines meant that my efforts were half-hearted. I had to change quite radically my attitude to and experience of working out in the gym in order to get the results that I wanted.

All habits begin with a single instance of a thought and then an action. Repeated over a lifetime they become hard to change. So how can we alter habitually negative behaviour? The answer is by being open to change, wanting to change, making a committed decision to change and then learning new positive behaviour patterns.

Now think about exercise habits that you may have learned. Are they positive or negative? Do you persevere with the same routine even though you don't get the results you want? Do you perform the same number of repetitions in an exercise even though it is no longer a challenge? Do you habitually procrastinate when it comes to fitness so that you don't get round to exercising at all. Think about the positive habits that you could develop instead.

Think about the type of habitual actions that would, for example, help you to work out consistently. How about putting your kit in your bag or car so that you can exercise at lunchtime or straight after work? Or try being flexible in your behaviour when you are no longer challenged: change the activity or the intensity so that you continue to get results.

Changing Your Behaviour

Our behaviour is the tip of the iceberg. Behind every 'behaviour' is an intention to achieve something of value to us. There is always a higher purpose. Now that might sound strange, especially if we think of our behaviour as negative and destructive. But whether your behaviour is empowering or limiting, the intention behind it is positive (don't worry, this will soon become clear).

So how do you get to the higher purpose behind your behaviour? You simply ask the question, 'What does this behaviour do for me?', wait for the answer and then ask the question again.

For example: 'What does avoiding exercise do for me?' 'It means that I don't have to make the effort.' And then, 'What does not making the effort do for me?' 'It makes me feel less stressed.' And finally, 'What does feeling less stressed do for me?' 'I am more relaxed. I enjoy life more.' Of course, wanting to feel relaxed is the positive intention (and something we would all like), but the value placed on effort means that a negative behaviour – avoiding exercise – is used to achieve that state of relaxation.

*Think
of a negative behaviour or habit that you
have in relation to exercise or activity. Write it down at
the top of your note pad. Now ask the question, 'What is my
positive intention behind this behaviour?' Trust the answers that
come out even if they seem illogical. If you don't come up
with a positive, put the answers underneath the
question then ask it again.*

Are you surprised at what you are finding? If your answers are not logical your unconscious mind is at work. Any answers that clash with your logical thinking are a symptom of something that is going on at a different level. When you find out the positive intention behind your behaviour you begin to open up your experience. And now, instead of fighting the behaviour that might or might not have served you well in the past, you find other ways to honour the intention behind it.

Sometimes we think that changing our behaviour will be hard or risky. You might feel a little apprehensive. What exactly will happen if I do change my behaviour? It is often easy to put off change because of a fear of the unknown. But it's worth repeating: if you always do what you have always done, you will always get what you always got in the past. In order to make changes in your life you need to do something different.

That something different does not have to be a hugely radical something. You could take a step-by-step approach so that you can monitor your progress as you develop a new attitude towards exercise and new behaviour. You simply need to be aware that although some behaviour is resistant to change, you do have a choice and you can change your behaviour if you really want to.

But how do we learn to develop new behaviour? We need to retrain our minds to change our thinking and the language that we use. We now know that by understanding the

The workout begins before you get to the gym.

higher purpose of your behaviour you are likely to be less resistant to change and able to make changes that honour that higher purpose. The exercises in this book will encourage you to do just that. We also need to move on to the next logical level of fitness to further fuel your motivation and empower you some more.

Capability

Just consider these statements: 'I can't do it', 'I am simply just not good at it' and 'I don't know how to do it.' If you find yourself using phrases such as these you clearly have misgivings about your capabilities. Sometimes people are challenged by having to learn new skills – and for physical fitness these new skills are essential. It's all very well having a positive mindset, but if you don't know how to put it to good use then you are not likely to get the results that you want from fitness, or you could develop poor exercise habits and pick up an injury. It is also important for your own confidence that you are doing the right things to reach your exercise goals. You will find an abundance of books and videos showing you 'How to ...', there are innumerable personal trainers and fitness instructors and health clubs with the latest gimmicks and gadgets. Aerobic pieces of equipment such as step, slide and spinning. For strength exercises there are stability balls, dynabands, free weights, rubber tubing and Ab curlers. For flexibility, yoga in all its different forms, and Pilate's for posture. The music at aerobics classes plays at exactly the right number of beats per minute. Instructors with high-tech microphone headsets boom out instructions. And yet, unfortunately, we have got it completely the wrong way round. We may have developed exercise to new levels of scientific efficiency, but we should really be focusing on what is happening on the inside, on the exerciser: the workout begins before you get to the gym.

Until recently we had no idea how to make the most of our mental resources and therefore put too much emphasis on physical training. But unless you have a positive mindset about fitness and exercise you are not likely to achieve your fitness goals. This is the feedback from that greater part of the population that is not exercising.

To achieve that positive mindset we need to focus on how to use the resources of the mind in the most effective way. The objective of this book is to encourage you to explore and then develop and hone your internal strategies, which will result in you becoming more skilful 'externally'.

When we first learn a skill we go through four stages. The first is unconscious incompetence. When you are unconsciously incompetent with regard to something, you have never tried, and therefore don't know how, to do that something. Where exercise is concerned, unconscious incompetence – not having exercised before – may mean that you have preconceived notions of what it is like. Perhaps you associate it with sport and, because you don't think of yourself as naturally sporty, have limiting beliefs about your self and your abilities. Because of this, some people don't even start exercising. Or you may believe that it will be too hard for you. However, if you do take the

Having never done a headstand, I managed to overcome my incompetance and finally achieve my objective.

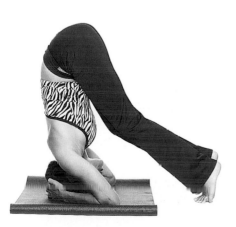
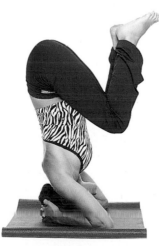

Think of a time when you were unconsciously competent at a given task, perhaps driving a car, riding a bike or typing. Remember what you did to get to that level of competence. How did you learn? Did you go through all of the stages above? Were you curious? Was the learning fun, exciting even? What resources did you use internally as well as externally?

Now think about your current exercise experience. What level of competence are you at? Is it worth you progressing to the next level? What internal and external resources do you need to get you to the next level? If you wanted to apply the resources that you used successfully to master a previous skill, how would you do so? Perhaps you simply need to be patient and allow yourself the time you need to improve.

But whatever our personal requirements, the thing we all need in order to become unconsciously competent at a given task is practice, practice, practice.

plunge – as of course you should – you will find yourself at the next stage: conscious incompetence.

When you are consciously incompetent you find that learning takes up a lot of your conscious attention. And you may feel a degree of apprehension and discomfort as you develop your new skills. (These feelings are exacerbated in those who are prone to self-consciousness.) In addition to this, our expectations of ourselves can be very high – we want results immediately and imagine that we will become experts in our chosen field overnight. At this stage the negative self-talk plays havoc, and we lose confidence if we don't feel we are progressing. This is very common in exercise classes. If an instructor sticks to the same routine then you will of course learn it over time. But if they change the routine every week, and especially if they introduce tricky moves, you may find yourself, unless you have exceptional co-ordination, stuck at this level. However, if you have the opportunity to practise enough at this level you will move on to the next: conscious competence.

Your beliefs can work for you or against you in life and they give meaning to your everyday behaviour.

When you are consciously competent you still have to think about what you are doing, but your ability to do it has improved enormously. At this level you will find that your confidence, self-esteem and sense of achievement grow in the exercise situation. You exercise more skilfully and this promotes positive behaviour. You are likely also to be progressing to a more general level of fitness and you are well on the way to the last logical level of learning, which is called unconscious competence.

When you are unconsciously competent your behaviour is 'automatic', streamlined and habitual. The subconscious part of your mind now directs your actions.

Beliefs

Our beliefs are the principles that guide our lives. They can remain constant or they can change over a lifetime – some are more deeply rooted than others. Many of our beliefs are likely to have been 'programmed' at an early age by those around us. This happens before our critical faculties have developed and while we are too young to question the beliefs we assimilate.

A belief is essentially any idea that you have accepted as true. When you accept a belief as true it becomes a generalization that will frame your thinking. What you believe about something will determine your attitude towards it, which then has an effect on your feelings and your actions. Your beliefs can work for you or against you in life and they give meaning to your everyday behaviour.

Beliefs have been described as the glue that holds your model of reality together. They underlie your thought patterns both conscious and unconscious, and they are a function of your programming whether that programming is right or wrong. Once you accept beliefs to be true you automatically act to make them true, and they establish boundaries to direct your future behaviour.

Your body will not do what your
mind does not believe it can.

Beliefs and Exercise

Of the limiting beliefs that prevent people from reaching their fitness
goals, one of the most common is 'I am not sporty.' This is likely to
be rooted in your past. If you aren't naturally sporty and repeatedly
had unpleasant experiences on the school playing fields,
negative associations may have developed into limiting
beliefs. And if you now associate exercise with sport, it
will trigger negative feelings towards the former.

Because we are all built differently, it *is* true that
some people are naturally more sporty than others.
But it is equally true – and more important – to say that
exercise is *not* sport. Sport is often highly competitive and team
based, demanding quite explosive movement. Exercise routines can
be devised for people of all abilities; it should be non-competitive
and you work at a pace that suits you. Health clubs are now
designed with both the sporty and the unsporty individual
in mind.

To change a limiting belief you need to challenge it. (If
you believe that you are not good at sport and exercise
then that is precisely what you will manifest. Your body
will not do what your mind does not believe it can.) You
do this by changing your perspective and finding other
ways to think about your belief. When you challenge your
old perspective you will find that it will lead to a new one.

Reference Experiences

Your beliefs are heavily influenced by your
experiences, both internally and externally.
For you to enjoy and be confident about
exercise you need to have positive internal
reference experiences. By creating external
reference experiences that are

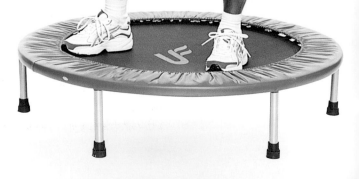

*Picture
an 'idea' as a tabletop without legs.
Whilst it is an idea there is nothing to support this
tabletop. As the idea forms and develops and you find the
reference experiences to back it up it becomes a belief. The
tabletop becomes supported by putting legs underneath
it. The more you can support the tabletop the
more solid the table becomes.*

achievable and making your exercise regime fun and 'do-able', you will build up positive internal reference experiences that will make you want to exercise again and again and again. Personal development Guru Anthony Robbins likened beliefs to tables. The exercise on this page shows you why.

Just imagine taking an exercise class for the first time. You have never exercised before and you are looking forward to it. You get started and find that you are completely uncoordinated and that the instructor is very difficult to follow. So you decide to try a step class instead. With the same result. Very soon your reference experience is one of failure.

I remember an experience while teaching exercise classes many years ago. Returning to the changing rooms, I would regularly see a powerful, athletic woman looking longingly into the classes. I spoke to her one day and thought that I would try to encourage her to go into the studio and have a go. But she completely lacked belief in herself and kept telling me that she would look an idiot if she actually attempted an exercise class. I found out that she had been an athlete in her youth and had won the 200 metres at many athletics meetings. We decided to have a few one-to-one sessions. This developed into two years of personal training. And when she finally did go into the studio there was no stopping her. No matter how powerful and sporty you may be, remember, your body will not do what your mind does not believe it can.

The reality is, of course, that everybody's motor skills are different. Some people can pick up new actions and movements easily, others take a little longer. But motor skills can vastly improve if you work at them. If you think you

*Just
imagine now how differently those
exercise sessions would be if you were to
wholeheartedly believe that you have the ability
to take on anything. Create an image in your
mind of you successfully
exercising.*

What are your current beliefs about exercise? Make a list of what you used to believe about physical activity, what you currently believe and what you want to believe in the future. What internal and external resources do you need to back up the belief you want to have?

are going to fall over your feet you will. But if you enter a class believing that you will learn, each time you go it will become easier and easier. You will develop positive internal reference experiences and fine tune your motor skills, which will enable you to get the most out of exercise classes.

Change Your Perspective

What did you find out when you did the mental exercises? Did you discover that your beliefs have changed over time or have they stayed the same? Is there an old belief that you want to discard so that you can move on? And do you feel that the belief that you want to have is achievable?

As long as you hold on to beliefs that limit you, you will find it hard to move forward. However, you can change your beliefs if you want to, and it isn't as difficult as you think. You just need to be ready to challenge yourself to find other ways to think about the situations you find yourself in. Remember, beliefs act as self-fulfilling prophecies. When we believe something to be true, we are likely to find that – consciously or otherwise – we make it true.

I remember a French lady who came to see me because she was suffering from depression. She had spent a lot of her childhood on her own and still felt desperately lonely. During one of our sessions she recalled something that her mother had said, 'Our sad little case, you will always be on your own.' Unfortunately, she believed her and to this day remained convinced that she was destined to be on her own. She needed to realize that she had to change what she believed about herself or that self-fulfilling prophecy would be with her for the rest of her life.

To prevent you falling victim to a self-fulfilling prophecy, here is an exercise adapted from NLP guru Robert Dilts's 'museum of old beliefs'.

Are there any self-fulfilling prophesies that affect you? Think about your experiences and jot them down. Here are some of the things that people say to themselves every day: 'I will never lose weight.' 'Every time I take that exam I know that I will fail it.' 'I will never find time to go to the gym.' 'My exercise goals will always be beyond me.'

Think of a belief that holds you back from reaching your fitness goals. For example, 'I am not sporty.' Now find at least three recent experiences that have proved this belief to be untrue. For example, 'I ran for a bus', 'I walked a good 30 minutes to work the other day', 'I played badminton in the garden with my children.'

Think of a useful belief that will replace the limiting one and open up new possibilities: 'Actually, I can see that I am able to become more physically active.'

Now imagine an image or a symbol for the old limiting belief. Imagine an old museum storage room, dark, dank and cobwebbed. Put the old belief in that room and then leave the museum.

Now create an image or symbol of the new helpful belief and imagine that you have placed it somewhere in your home where you will see it all the time. Decide that every time you look at it that you will be even more empowered by your new belief.

Values

Your values determine what is important to you. They can demotivate you or fuel your motivation and set the course of action for your future. Your values determine the standards by which you judge yourself and the rest of the world. For example, if what you value most in life is wealth, then you will probably find yourself thinking about the financial implications of every decision you make. You may judge your success – or lack thereof – in terms of money, and you may even reject people who do not have the same values as you. If good health is high on your list of values then regular exercise, eating properly and a good night's sleep will be important to you. The values we hold are hierarchical, with some higher than others on our list of priorities. If, for example, you value wealth above health, you will do that extra hour of overtime instead of your planned session at the gym.

Core Values

Sometimes what you say has what is called a 'surface value'. These are supported by other values. In other words, the values behind the values. These core values influence you at an unconscious level. When you are aware of your core values, you have a better understanding of what is motivating or demotivating you.

Think of something you value and ask yourself the following questions in order to find your core value. For example, 'What do you value about this thing?' 'It makes me feel good.' And then, 'What do you value about feeling good?' I'm more confident in my dealings with the world.' Finally, 'What do you value about being more confident?' 'I feel at peace with myself.'

What about exercise? Do you value it? What do you value about it? What do you not value? Make a list of both and then compare them. Now write a list of ways in which you could value every part of the exercise process. Explore the areas you do not value and allow your personal coach to talk to you through them.

Take a moment and close your eyes. Imagine a movie screen with a picture of you on it. Imagine what you will look like in five years' time if you don't exercise. Take a good look and then blank the screen. Now imagine what you will look like in ten years' time if you don't exercise. Take a good look and then blank the screen. Now imagine what you will look like in 30 years' time if you don't exercise. If you don't like what you've seen and want to picture a healthier, fitter you, then mark this exercise with a resounding tick.

Most people value a fitter, healthier body but not the effort and discomfort it will take to get it. By recognizing the true value of exercise, by recognizing the benefits it will bring, you will be encouraged to get beyond the negative thoughts you may have had in the past.

Unfortunately, we often value exercise only when our health suffers. For example, if we develop heart problems or become dangerously overweight. Then the fundamental desire to get better and live longer – core values if ever there were any – motivate us to exercise.

Identity

If you have heard someone say 'I am not sporty' or 'That is just not me', you are hearing a statement that reveals that person's perception of their identity. Identity is a question of who you think you are. We can have a number of identities in our lifetimes – some are permanent, others are not.

Our identities are what we feel ourselves to be most essentially in life. But even this can change. Think how a mother's identity is challenged as her children leave home. Or if you were to move from one country to another, how your cultural identity would be challenged. (My father is Jamaican. Although he has lived in England for over 40 years he still has a strong accent and insists on having Caribbean food for lunch on Sunday. When asked who he is, he responds with 'I am a Jamaican.' These are his ways of holding on to his cultural identity.)

It is important when establishing your identity to separate who you are from what you do. Your behaviour is not your identity. Take, for example, this statement: 'I was told at school that I wasn't very good at sport, so I

Think of the number of identities that you have. My own, for example, would include 'I am fit', 'I am a mother', 'I am of mixed race', 'I am a spiritual person.'

know I'm not sporty, and therefore I'm not going to exercise.' 'I'm not sporty' – this person has confused their behaviour and limiting beliefs with their identity (and made the old mistake of associating exercise with sport).

A young horsewoman came to see me because she wanted to ride with more confidence. As we talked I discovered that every time she went to her riding lessons both her teacher and her father would be there giving her lots of 'useful advice'. She felt completely smothered and her faith in herself had been shaken. She had been taking the criticism personally and was beginning to lose her sense of self. A very useful tool for her was to understand that they were talking about her skills and her behaviour and not about who she was. She had to learn to separate the two. Once she could differentiate between self and behaviour, her confidence began to grow. She could become more objective about her abilities and not take the 'advice' personally.

A colleague of mine gave a wonderful example: 'I am a spiritual being on a physical journey.' Needless to say, he chose yoga with its dual emphasis on meditation and movement.

Take a moment to think about yourself. Ask yourself 'Who am I?' Jot down what pops into your mind. Now go on asking yourself 'Who else am I?' until you exhaust the question. Now take the list and read it to yourself and after each identity say to yourself 'Yes, and I am more than that.' Be aware of your feelings as you do so. Do you enjoy stepping beyond those labels? Do you feel a sense of possibility and opening? Now look at the list and choose one label that you like the best. What kind of exercise regime would suit that label?

*Spend
a few moments with pen and paper in
hand. Focus on your breathing – allow yourself to relax
and dream. Do you have any dreams that are yet to be realized?
As you look back on your life, is there a pattern that tells you about
the path that you are taking, your mission? Where are you now on that
path? Do you have a strong sense of purpose, of knowing where
you are going? Imagine yourself in old age looking back at
yourself and ask yourself 'Have I achieved my
purpose in life?'*

Beyond Identity

This is the point at which we embrace the concept of oneness with the
universe, a recognition that we are part of a larger system. For some this
is a spiritual truth or related to a belief in God or gods. For others it is
simply a question of seeing the bigger picture. Jeffery Hodges, in his
book *Champion Feeling*, suggests that we are not just products of
past socialization and conditioning but that we are a 'pre-sequence of
our future'. It is having a dream, a vision, a real sense of purpose that will
allow us to 'realize' and develop that future self, enabling us to grow into
our full potential and leading to states of fulfilment and satisfaction and
happiness. Individuals who have a strong sense of mission are more
purposeful, more likely to be successful in life and are more fulfilled.
People who have no sense of purpose tend to wander aimlessly through
life with a sense of underachievement, feelings of unfulfilment and more
depressed states of mind.

Here is how I understand my own life. I have a very strong sense of a
mission to help others be the best they can be. As I realize my own
potential I can pass on my knowledge to others. The discovery that we
have the most incredible resources within us to achieve our lives' missions
has been the most enlightening experience of my lifetime. With this
enlightenment I have reached states of well-being and happiness that I
never thought possible. Hoping to help others through my own
experiences, as I take myself forward to the end of my lifetime I have a
real sense that I have accomplished this vision to the best of my ability.

Individuals who have a strong sense of mission are more purposeful, more likely to be successful in life and are higher achievers.

How does exercise fit into this 'life mission'? What are the benefits it will bring? How would a strong, fit body help with this purpose? How would being less stressed help? Or having bundles of energy and vitality? What kinds of exercise would fit in with this sense of purpose – a good walk to be at one with nature, an aerobics class to connect with others, yoga postures to induce a sense of peace and calm?

Levels of Change

Each of the levels we have just explored interrelates with the others. If one level changes then you are likely see change on the others. If, for example, you change a limiting belief from 'I can't ...' to 'I can ...', it is likely to affect your sense of who you are and your capabilities and, ultimately, your attitude and behaviour.

At what level do you think you need to begin the process of change? Is it your environment that you need to change – the place and time for exercise? Perhaps it is your behaviour that needs to be adjusted. How are your fitness skills? What level of competence are you at and what do you need to work on? What do you believe now? Do you need to change your beliefs? How can you value exercise more highly so that you do it consistently? You may look at your existing exercise regime and ask, 'Is this me?', 'Does this enhance who I am?', 'How does exercise fit into my bigger picture?'

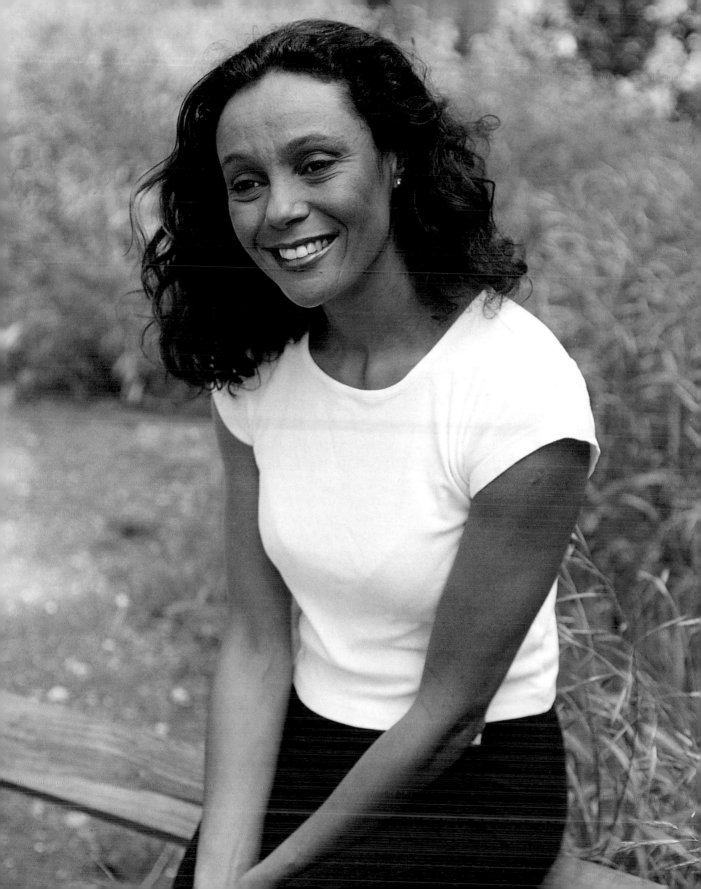

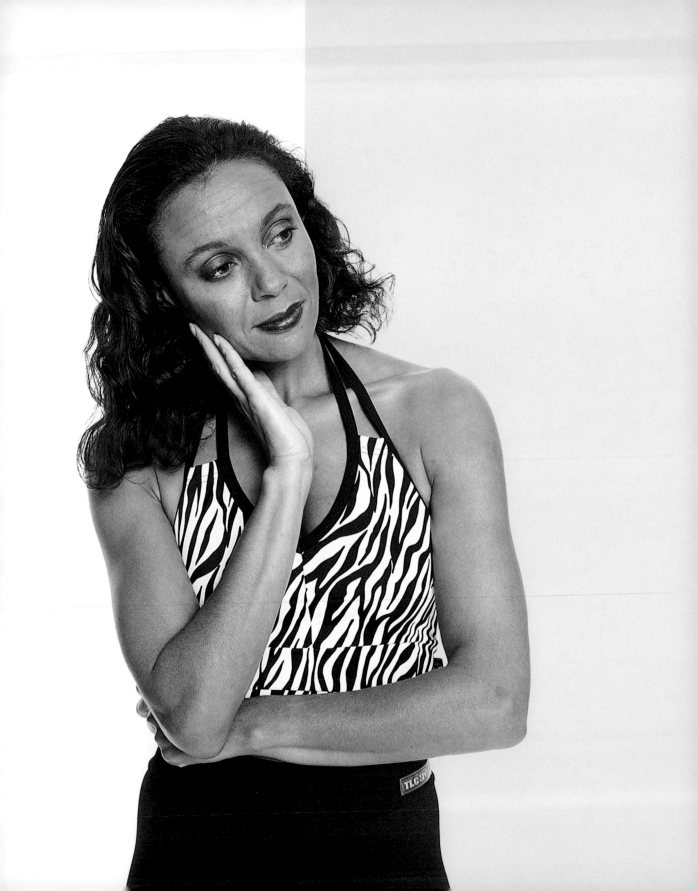

Chapter 5

Setting Your Goals

Positive motivation is the force that will get you getting fit. Negative motivation will also enable you to do it, but the process is likely to be more difficult. But what is the point of being motivated if you don't know your end goal. You say you want to get fit, fit for what?

Setting Your Goals

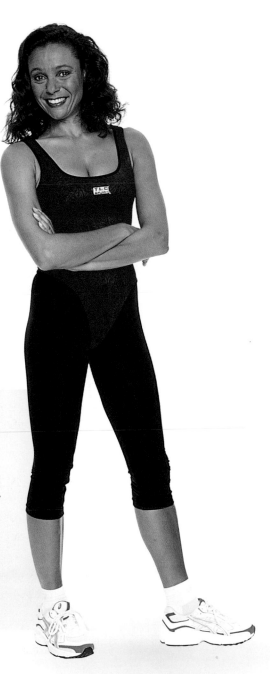

The mind has been described as a heat-seeking missile and one of its prime functions is to work towards the goals it is given. We make goals in our minds all the time even though we might not be aware of it. (Quite often people don't know what they want, though they may know very well what they don't want.) We are always working towards something. Everything that we do has a reason behind it, whether it is pruning the roses, passing an examination or dropping a few kilos in weight. A goal will take you from where you are now to where you want to be, and the more specific you can be about what you want, the more likely you are to get it.

So what is your exercise goal? Well, here is a list of the reasons other people give for wanting to get fit. Add your own to the list.

- To look better
- To feel better
- To function better
- To get into my clothes
- For greater energy and vitality
- To be healthier
- To combat stress
- To be more confident
- To have a postive self image

Add your own

Although some of us suffer from resistance to exercise we want the benefits it brings. Just think – you will look better, you will feel better, and exercise fights stress. It helps women maintain weight during pregnancy and has been associated with a better delivery. For chaps, exercise helps to keep testosterone levels high and combats abdominal obesity, which increases the risk of heart disease. It also combats conditions such as osteoporosis, cardiovascular disease, diabetes and depression, to name but a few. In fact, go to the doctor's surgery nowadays and you may get a prescription for exercise. It is great for the skin and rids the body of toxins, and it will allow you to achieve your best body shape. You look younger and have more energy and vitality. The body pumps feel-good hormones into your system. The list is (almost) endless.

When you know what you want from exercise you are ready to begin – definite goals suggest specific solutions. But beware: often we focus on what we don't want and we all too often get it. If, for example, you keep telling yourself 'I'm so unfit' and 'Oh no, I'm getting fatter and fatter', you could be directing your subconscious mind to 'achieve' just that. Your subconscious mind does not discriminate between positive and negative. It simply works towards the suggestions you give it and the result in this case is that you stay fat and unfit.

Why Don't People Reach Their Goals?

Some people don't set goals for fear of failure – or even of what life might be like if they were successful. We are often afraid of the feedback that we get from the outside world. Other people can dampen your enthusiasm with negative comments or simply by persuading you to do something else. You may find that you have a day when other priorities get in the way. Instead of getting back on course and simply accepting that you have had a bad day, you spiral into decline, feel that you have failed miserably and give up for good.

There is no such thing as failure, only feedback.

Consider the stories of some very successful people. Colonel Saunders Kentucky, the fried-chicken king, took his recipes to 1009 restaurants and food outlets before any interest was shown. It took Thomas Edison thousands of attempts before he invented a light bulb that worked. When asked how it felt to have failed so many times, Edison answered that he hadn't failed at all, but rather he had successfully found thousands of ways of not inventing the light bulb!

These people found the way to achieve their goals: they never gave up despite the negative feedback. They recognized that there are no failures, only experiences that we can learn from in order to find the right way to succeed. They believed in themselves.

If you have not enjoyed exercise in the past in may mean that the feedback that you get from exercise was physically, mentally and emotionally uncomfortable. As I mentioned before, all human behaviour is influenced by what is painful or pleasurable, and an essential resource for thinking yourself fit is to ensure that you get positive feedback from your exercise experience. If you evaluate your feedback in a constructive way and you can perceive the experience of exercise to be less challenging and more pleasurable, you are more likely to achieve your goals.

So what else might have prevented you from reaching your goals in the past? Well, perhaps you left them to chance or relied on external resources. Or you simply didn't know how to go about reaching them. Do you set yourself 'big' goals and then become caught up in the challenge they present? Perhaps you have used negative language to talk yourself out of exercise. Are you inflexible in your behaviour, focusing on only one way of reaching your goals? (In fact, the more flexible you are and the more choice you allow yourself, the more likely you are to be successful.) Perhaps your goals have been at odds with who you are (remember our logical levels of fitness).

Think of an experience that you had of exercising or making the decision to exercise. Were you focusing on how well you were doing or were you beating yourself up and talking yourself out of (potential) discomfort. As you relive this situation do you have a sense of being on the inside looking out or outside, as an observer looking in? If the former, step out of yourself by imagining that you are in your front room watching a video of yourself on the telly and that you are in charge of the remote control.

As you watch your experience on the telly, play around with the remote control to change the colours on the screen and the volume and perhaps the language that you are using. Begin to change your own responses to the situation. Enhance the experience if it is positive and change it if it is negative. What would you want to feel? What would you like to hear yourself say? What actions would you be taking?

Think now of resources and feelings that might be useful for you to fully change that experience: confidence, perhaps, self-belief or a sense of calm. Remember a time when you had these resources. Relive the experience. Then imagine you are bringing these resources to that experience. When you have tuned in the resources you need to make sure that the picture is perfect for you, so fiddle with the controls until you get it just right. Press the play button and watch the movie of your experience. Notice how it differs from the 'original'.

Now blank the screen. Imagine a time in the future when you find yourself in a similar situation, which in the past would have caused you discomfort. Again, be aware of the differences in what you see, hear and feel. Imagine stepping into the picture now and trying your 'role' on for size. The result should be a very positive experience. But if you feel that you need further resources, go back until the experience feels, looks and sounds just as you want it to.

Write down a goal that you want to achieve and list all the skills you will need. Now ask yourself the question, 'What is the obstacle that stops me reaching this goal?' Is it procrastination, your limiting beliefs, laziness, or that the task is too big? Identify which of them is the real 'obstacle'.

Ask yourself, 'If this obstacle was not there, would I be able to move forward and reach my goal?' Yes or no? If the answer is 'no', you need to ask yourself what other other obstacles are in your way?

Ask yourself if these obstacles were not there would you be able to move forward? If your goal is to exercise in the park for 30 minutes every day, then the obstacle may be: 'I will look silly exercising in the park.'

Identify at least three ways to remove the obstacle. Firstly, decide that you won't do anything that will make you look too odd – you can do your warming up and stretching at home. Secondly, choose an exercise such as power walking or gentle jogging that won't draw attention to you. Finally, decide to work at a pace that is not too challenging – one that won't leave you red-faced, sweat soaked and looking as though you are on the point of collapse.

You need some bright pens and crayons, a few sheets of blank paper and ten minutes without interruption. The exercise below draws on a technique called clustering. It is a brainstorming process that gets your thoughts out of your head and onto paper. So just write down what you want out of exercise.

A mind map showing a brainstorm that explores how to function better.

FUNCTION BETTER

Natural high
Focus
Better circulation
Reduce toxins
Sweat
Chemical changes
Improved lungs
Heart
Concentrate
Feel FAB
Great confidence
Strong muscles
Organs
Bendy body
Effort
Feel well
Endurance
Patience
Pace
Look good
Feel confident

Take one of your exercise goals from the exercise on the opposite page and ask, 'What will that do for me?' Repeat the question until you can go no further. For example, 'I want to tone my muscles.' 'What will that do for me?' 'It will make me a stronger person.' 'What will that do for me?' 'I will have a stronger face to show the world.' 'What will that do for me?' 'I will feel able to accept more challenges.' 'What will that do for me?' 'It will give me a sense of fulfilment.'

Having a clear sensory experience of your goal and the process that you will be going through to reach it will fuel your desire and will-power.

Using Your Senses

The next question is how do you know that you have reached or are reaching your goal? Often we set a goal and start working towards it but are not aware of changes that are taking place, or we do not recognize our successes along the way. This can result in feelings of failure, in negative inner dialogue, and result in drop-out. Having a clear sensory experience of your goal and the process that you will be going through to reach it will fuel your desire and will-power. To let you know that you are moving towards it or you have successfully achieved it, practice using your senses.

The next time you have a bath or a shower, take a good look at yourself in the mirror and observe your curves, your contours. Talk out loud to yourself about what you see and listen to what you hear yourself saying. Take your awareness now to how you feel. Are you pleased with what you see or is there a sense of dissatisfaction? Pay close attention to your experience.

Now do the same thing with your eyes shut. Recreate what you just saw, heard and felt. Bring it all back – the picture, sounds and feelings – as vividly as you can.

If you have followed the exercise on this page, you will see that we have the most amazing inner world. It is made up of our visual (seeing), auditory (hearing), kinaesthetic (feeling), gustatory (tasting) and olfactory (smelling) senses. The three that are most useful for fuelling your motivation and setting goals for fitness are your visual, auditory and kinaesthetic senses. Everything that we have ever experienced in our lifetimes is stored in the subconscious mind ready to be brought back to us through those sensory channels. Most of us have a sense that is more powerful than the others, and there are a number of ways to find out which yours is.

Visual

If you are predominately visual then you are probably motivated to exercise to look good and you will be influenced by what you see. So an exercise environment that is pleasing to the eye will be important to you. A studio with mirrors or a well-designed health club will help; grubby mats and finger marks on mirrors might be off putting. If you are taking a class, the way the instructor looks may be important to you, providing a role model for you to copy. You are disposed toward thinking in images, so you will learn best by imitating an instructor or working with a visually interesting book or video, or by watching something entertaining while you're on the treadmill.

Auditory

If you are predominately auditory you are primarily motivated by what you hear. So a teacher who verbalizes instructions clearly will be important, as will tone of voice and the right kind of music. Music can be used in any situation to boost your mood, which will help you to enjoy exercise (although the wrong music will bore the pants off you). If your auditory sense is weak, you may not be aware of your internal dialogue.

Kinaesthetic

If you are predominantly kinaesthetic you will have a more refined sense of body awareness and you will be influenced by how you feel. So the type of exercise you choose will be important to you. You may also feel inclined to exercise in an environment in which you feel comfortable – too hot or too cold, for example, could put you off. It might pay for you to get fit with a friend so that you can share a sense of 'feel-good' while you work out.

Your Language

You can also tell which sensory system is predominant by examining the language you use. If you litter your talk with sensory phrases such as 'That looks great', 'Seeing is believing' and 'I can't say until I've seen it', you are probably a visual person. You may be drawn to media such as movies or the visual arts. An auditory person uses language that relates to sound, 'That sounds great', 'I hear what you are saying', 'This is music to my ears', and is drawn to music, the radio and reading. A kinaesthetic person is likely to say things such as 'That feels right' and 'He is a pain in the neck' and to lean towards leisurely activities such as massage or a form of alternative therapy.

A Sensory Questionnaire

The following exercise will determine which is your dominant sense. By discovering your dominant sense you will know what is most likely to motivate you and you will also be able to focus your attention on your weaker senses and make them stronger.

Add up the 'v's (for 'visual'), 'k's (for 'kinaesthetic') and 'a's (for 'auditory'). Obviously, the more there are of any one, the greater the extent to which that sensory system predominates. If you find that they are more or less equal, it may mean that you have an equal balance or simply that further work needs to done to uncover your strongest sense

I develop exercise skills most effectively by
- practising the actions (k)
- listening to instructions from a coach (a)
- seeing the exercises performed (v)

I am most motivated to exercise by
- stimulating music (a)
- the thought of how I am going to look (v)
- knowing that I will feel good (k)

I am most drawn to an exercise environment
- that is pleasing to the eye (v)
- offers expert coaching advice (a)
- in which I feel comfortable (k)

The decisions that I make about exercise are determined by
- my gut reaction (k)
- the information I hear (a)
- what I see (v)

I prefer to
- listen to music or the radio (a)
- watch the television or see a movie (v)
- do something physically active or have a massage (k)

If I were taking a walk by a river, I'd prefer to
- enjoy the scenery around me (v)
- play music on my walkman as I go (a)
- focus on how I'm feeling (k)

When I'm familiar with an exercise
- I can explain how it's done to other people (a)
- I have a clear picture in my mind of what I have to do (v)
- I find practising it easy (k)

I am more easily motivated by
- a clear image in my mind of what I want (v)
- positive self-talk (a)
- how good something makes me feel (k)

I most often think in
- pictures (v)
- sounds (a)
- I go by how I feel (k)

I plan my goals by
- picturing them in my mind (v)
- verbalizing what I need to do (a)
- knowing how I am going to feel (k)

I am most influenced to exercise by
- The way I look (v)
- The words I use (a)
- The way I feel (k)

I communicate what is going on with me through
- the feelings I share (k)
- the words I choose (a)
- how I look (v)

You can do this exercise with your eyes open or closed – what is important is that you relax. You can do this by spending a moment or two focusing on your breathing. Now allow yourself to dream. Imagine that in front of you is a giant movie screen and on it is an image of you as you wish to be. For example, 'My muscles look tight and toned and I see myself looking relaxed and happy.' What will you be hearing when you reach this goal? ' I hear others saying how great I look and a positive dialogue within me.' What will you be feeling? 'I will be feeling strong, centred, focused and relaxed.'

When you have worked out your dominant sense you can exploit it to help you learn how to get fit. You can enhance it and/or make your weaker senses stronger. For example, a visual person may want to explore their kinaesthetic sense by practising body awareness, which means being more in tune with your body and aware of how exercise makes you feel – the main determiner of our actions. An auditory person could develop a stronger visual sense by practicing visualization. A kinaesthetic person could develop auditory skills by choosing motivating music to work out to, music that stimulates them to exercise for longer and takes away inhibitions. You can also use music to pace your exercise.

Each of these senses can be used as a powerful tool for learning in every area of life. If what you want to do is get fit, you create a positive image of how you want to look, use your auditory skills to talk yourself into position and your kinaesthetic skills to monitor and control how you feel. It is now time to use your senses to motivate you and even reprogramme your thought processes to enable you to move towards your fitness goal.

It is now time to use your senses to motivate you and even reprogramme your thought processes to enable you to move towards your fitness goal.

Motivators

Here are some tips to help you make the most of your senses. If you're a visual person, wear some snazzy kit, choose a realistic model to aspire to, visualize your goals in the morning and evening and set them so that you measure your progress, perhaps by taking measurements (of your chest, waist, hips, thighs). While you are on the treadmill watch television.

If your auditory sense predominates, use a walkman to stimulate you while you work out, coach yourself through your exercise by talking to yourself – make sure your inner trainer is giving you positive feedback – and use motivating music to psych you up.

If you are kinaesthetic, wear exercise gear and shoes that feel comfortable, stay aware of how good exercise makes you feel and choose a variety of activities that you feel comfortable with.

A positive visual, auditory or kinaesthetic experience will fuel motivation and guide your mind to work towards your goal. As you inevitably experience resistance on the way, you can guide and take control of your sensory skills. You can begin the process of changing negative programming to positive in order to further motivate you towards your fitness goals.

The next question is: when you have planned and set your goal, will you be able to maintain your efforts to achieve it?

If you're a visual person, wear some snazzy kit to motivate you to reach your goal.

Self-Maintained

Perhaps one of the biggest challenges on the way to getting fit is achieving consistency, the lack of which can often result in drop-out. Think of what happens in January or February. You come out of hibernation and join a gym or start to exercise at home after the excesses of Christmas. You keep going for a month or so and then something else seems to happen and you find yourself rushing home from work with a Chinese takeaway and a video! (If you joined a gym, just think of the money you've wasted – a year's subscription for a handful of sessions!)

All kinds of things may be happening here. As you achieve your goals you may find yourself demotivated and directionless – a new ambition is needed to keep you going. Perhaps you were overwhelmed by the goal you set yourself – or it was too small and not challenging enough. Or you find that you do not reach your goals because you are too dependent on factors outside your control. It could be the weather, a babysitter or a friend who is an unreliable exercise partner. Perhaps not getting the results you wanted quickly enough is all it takes to make you want to give it up.

If achieving your fitness goal relies on external factors, you may be making your task more difficult for yourself. Is there a way of sidestepping them?

It is when you find your motivation wavering that you really need to work on it. Make the task of exercise as easy as possible. Constantly remind yourself of the benefits so that you continue to value exercise. Reinforce your committed decision to exercise and the goals that you are now developing in your mind. Really believe that you can do it. This is what you need to do to guarantee success.

Now that you know what you want from fitness and have a clear sensory experience of it in your mind, we can look at the basic principles of goal setting and other ways to maintain your goal.

Does your goal rely on external factors? If the answer is yes then you may be making the task more difficult for yourself. Are there other ways you can achieve your outcome allowing yourself to let go of the need for external influences?

Your goals should fit in with your life and your life should fit in with your goals.

It is important to be realistic about your shape and accept it and then work out what you will have to do to get the best body you can.

S.M.A.R.T.

SPECIFIC: we have already said that in order to be successful with a goal it is essential to know what you want. The more specific you can be about what you have to do and how you are going to do it, the more chance you have of getting there. If you are a member of a gym, work with a fitness instructor to set up an exercise regime specific to your goal, time requirements and capabilities. If you're not a gym member, read up on your particular area of interest. Explore how often you need to exercise, how hard you need to work, how long you need to exercise for. Devise a weekly timetable for exercise and pin it up on your fridge door. If you want to measure your fitness levels, try a step test, take your pulse or do the talk test. The easiest method is the talk test. If, when you are exercising, you can talk easily you are not working hard enough. If you are completely out of breath then you are working too hard. If you can hold a breathy conversation then you are working at the right level. If your goal is to get into a dress or a pair of trousers that haven't fitted you for years, how many inches do you need to lose? Monitor your progress by taking regular measurements or simply keep trying the clothes on until you can get into them. Your timetable may be disrupted every week, but if you plan ahead as much as possible and change the time at which you exercise rather than cancelling completely, you are more likely to succeed.

MEANINGFUL: set goals that can be self-maintained by you.

ACHIEVABLE: it is essential that you set goals that you will be able to achieve. You may need professional advice to gauge your fitness abilities and draw up your physical fitness programme. But perhaps even more importantly, you need to focus on what is achievable mentally and emotionally. You need to accept that you may have limitations and then work within them. For example, if you have only two windows in your schedule for exercise and it is impossible to fit in any more, then those two sessions are better than none! Acknowledge that it may take longer to get the results you want.

You may have unrealistically high expectations of your body type. The media bombards us with images of the 'ideal' body shape for us to emulate. But the supermodel look is not achievable for many – let alone everyone. It is important to be realistic about your shape and accept it and then work out what you will have to do to get the best body you can.

You might have been sporty at school but are you still? If you have not exercised for many years, are you realistic about your abilities now? Recently, an overweight 40-year-old man came to see me because he could no longer play football at the level he used to. He was trying so hard to keep up that all he was doing was picking up injuries. I assured him that he could play football again, but he should train first. He had to recognize that his body had very particular needs.

REVIEW: your goals: you need regular goal checks so that you can see yourself progress. Be aware of where you have come from and where you are now – this will fuel your motivation and strengthen your resolve for the future. Focus on positive reference experiences to keep you going. Some people who come to see me are despondent because they aren't reaching their goals quickly enough. I tell them that it has taken many years to get themselves into the condition – good or bad – that they are in now. Nothing happens to the body overnight – certainly not miracles. I then ask them to make a list of what has worked for them in the past. Focus on what is working rather that what is not working.

TIME: it is important to give yourself a realistic time frame in which to achieve your goals. If you are unfit and you set a six-month time frame to train to run the London Marathon, do you think you'll be successful? Imagine the stress that you would be putting yourself under to reach that goal. Equally, if you set a goal and give yourself too much time, you may lose motivation along the way. Are you consistently giving yourself ten minutes a day to do your mind exercises? Have you established a regular routine, setting aside certain times of the day, that you can easily stick to?

Remind youself of these simple principles and to tell yourself that you are a SMART exerciser and well on the way to success.

Ecology

Finally, when you set a goal you need to be sure that you will be able to achieve it as effortlessly as possible taking into consideration all the aspects of life that are important to you. If there is any resistance in your life, it is likely to affect the decisions you make about exercise. So ask yourself 'Is it worth doing?' How will working toward your goal affect the other people in your life? If you spend all your time at the gym, how will this affect your relationships elsewhere? Will your partner mind? Is it worth the time and effort it is going to take? Realistically, how much time and effort will it take? Will you have to give anything up to reach this outcome? If so, is it worth it?

How far have you progressed since you started your exercise regime? What has worked so far? Make a list of positive reference experiences of mental, emotional and physical changes. Which of those experiences will be useful for the future? How is the fine-tuning of your senses coming along? Are you now more aware of your internal dialogue and the pictures that you make in your mind? How is your body awareness? What level of competence are you at now? Are you still as committed as before? With all of this in mind, what is the next step for you?

*Imagine
what it will take to achieve your
fitness goals. How will this affect other areas of
your life – your work, your home life, your friends, your
personal development and the other things that you
value? If there are any conflicts, make adjustments
so that your goal and your life meet
halfway.*

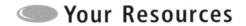 ## Your Resources

How do you set a goal that is achievable? You do so by creating a realistic framework that you know you will enable you to achieve that end result. You then find the resources, both internal and external, that will help you reach that goal. In the past you may have focused too much on external resources – the latest fitness fads, such as step, slide, Tai Bo, which are all supposed to make exercise easier or more efficient. While external resources are very useful, it is our internal resources that are really going to make the difference to our attempts to get fit. Indeed to our success in life.

But when setting yourself a goal, you need to be really clear about exactly what it is that you want. When you know what you want, you will begin to feel an invisible force pulling you towards your goal. So what *do* you want?

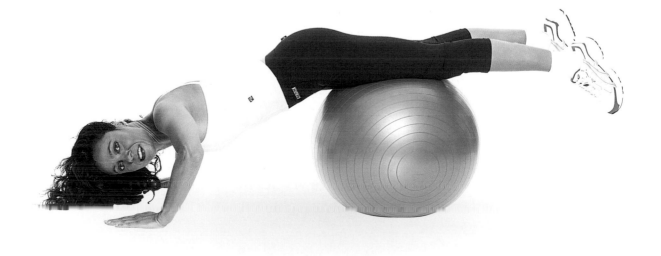

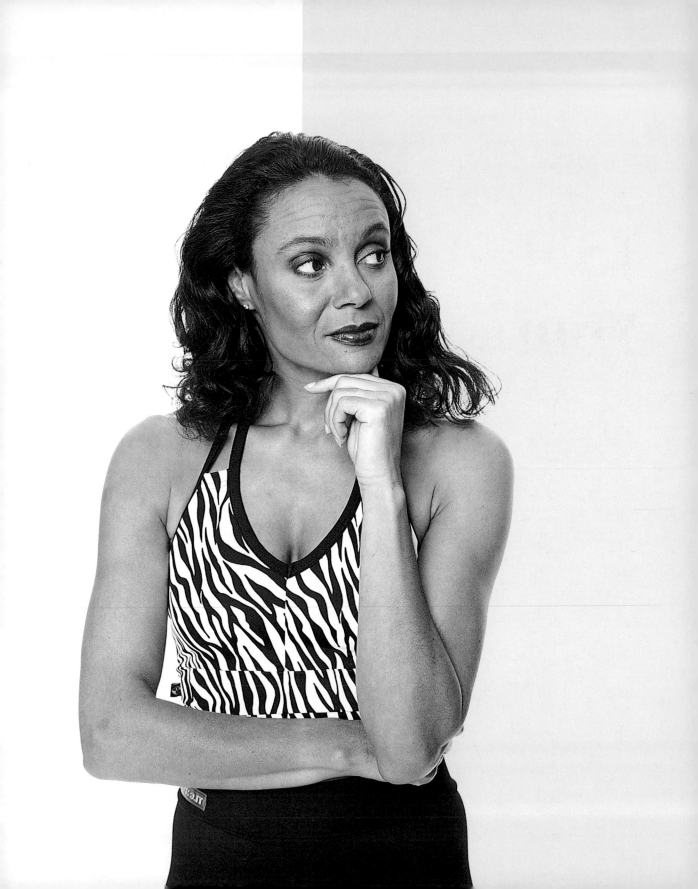

Chapter 6

Tools to Think Yourself Fit

What else do you need in order to change the conditioning of a lifetime? You must now be aware that you have the resources within you to achieve what you want from fitness, to be your own personal trainer and coach yourself to success. When you set your goal for fitness you discovered the three senses to utilize: visual, auditory and kinaesthetic. You discovered how we use these senses all the time even though we may not be aware of it. Now you are more consciously aware you can use your senses to make changes in your life, to work towards your goals, to talk yourself through any resistance you may come up against and to challenge any negative internal dialogue.

Tools to Think Yourself Fit

When you next exercise be aware of what you are saying to yourself and even write it down. I often have a laugh at the verbal batterings I give myself. Are you being kind to yourself or are you beating yourself up? If you were a personal trainer, what kinds of thing would you say to a client to motivate, encourage and even counsel them.

Association and Disassociation

Another way to move towards your goals and ensure you get positive feedback is to change your perception of the physical side of exercise. If you 'associate into' how you are feeling you can be put off by the challenge or discomfort of exercise. I remember taking a client running. She kept on puffing and panting and telling me how awful it felt. I had to find ways to distract her, and when she took the attention away from herself she found that time just flew by. As we associate into the experience of exercise, our perception of it can be distorted. In other words, in your mind you make it a more uncomfortable experience than it really is.

So when you are associated you look out through your own eyes, you are aware of your feelings and sensations, and your language suggests that you are 'in' the experience. And when you are disassociated you have a sense of distance from your body, you are much less aware of your feelings and sensations, and your voice is likely to be more monotone than usual.

You need to know that you can change your experience by simply acknowledging your tendency to exaggerate and by finding ways to distract yourself. This will ensure that you don't get caught up in the physical feelings of activity. It is important to associate into the feelings of exercise when you start to learn about correct technique and how to monitor the intensity of your workout. But once you know what you are doing you can find ways to distance yourself from the experience so that it becomes more tolerable if not pleasurable.

Think of the feedback you get about exercise before doing it or actually while exercising, for example, 'it is too much effort to get to the gym tonight' or 'this is too hard for me'. As you revisit this experience do you have a sense of being back in the experience as if you were really there? Or are you looking on from an observer's position? Note what you see, hear and feel.

If you are back in the experience as if you were really there you will have a sense of actually feeling the experience. If you are observing the experience as an onlooker you will find that you may not be getting much feeling from the experience.

Have a go at swapping the two around. If you are associated with the experience just see yourself stepping out of it and taking the place of the onlooker. If you are more disassociated, step into the experience and fully experience what you see hear and feel.

Here are some more suggestions to help you move your attention away from exercise when you need to.

- Great music will take your mind off what you are doing, stimulate you and keep you going for longer. If you are going to join a health club, try to make sure the teachers have the sort of music collection that will give you the boost you need.
- A distracting environment will mean that you can get lost in what you see around you.
- Exercise with a friend so that you can gossip away and lose track of time.
- Run your own movie in your own head or dream about life and things that you want.
- If you are working out on a bicycle or treadmill, make sure there are television screens in front of you so that you can trance out while you watch something you really like. (I can easily do 60 minutes if *The Bill* is on!)
- If you are exercising at home, have a collection of your favourite videos to hand or tape something interesting and save it for your exercise session.
- Use a personal stereo to listen to while you power walk.
- If you have a problem that needs solving, make an agreement with yourself to put it out of your mind until you have finished your exercise. Then, as you exercise, allow yourself to dream. You'll be amazed how easily problems can be solved when you approach them with a fresh mind.
- Step back from any negative feedback or dialogue that you may be hearing from those around you or that you might create yourself.

So do you tend to associate fully into your exercise experience or do you disassociate more? How can you apply these techniques to your own exercise regime or to your thinking about fitness? Which would be more useful to you?

Relaxation

You might have noticed that in most of the exercises I have encouraged you to work with a relaxed frame of mind. It is this relaxed state that will allow you to take control of your own mind easily and effortlessly. Relaxation is the gentle art of being able to control your thinking and the gateway to your inner mind. It is amazing that we have this incredibly simple tool but have never really made good use of it. When the mind is relaxed you receive the most incredible physical benefits – blood pressure drops, heart and breathing rate slow so that oxygen consumption decreases by 20 per cent, muscle tension decreases, the flow of blood to the extremities increases – and you experience a wonderful sense of well-being as energy flows through your body and mind.

Enhanced Perception

As your body relaxes so does your mind, enhancing your perception and heightening your awareness. You may find that in this state problems are easier to solve and your creativity is increased. Relaxing allows you to be aware of your magical inner world and that awareness allows you to make changes where needed. It also creates harmony between both body and mind and frees up your thoughts. In this state of relaxation you quieten the conscious mind and allow the subconscious mind to become dominant. Most sports psychologists recommend relaxation with mental imagery training. When the mind is relaxed it is free of clutter, which enables you then to focus on what you really want instead. Suggestions and images can be placed in the subconscious mind, which is now more likely to accept them. It's a great alternative to logical thought.

Relaxing is not the same as going to sleep or other so-called restful activities such as having a cup of tea or slumping in front of the television. Sleep, in fact, can be very active and emotional. If you practise relaxation before sleeping it will improve the quality of your sleep. And if you are an insomniac, practise relaxation when you can't sleep and you will get

Sit in a comfortable position and take a few deep breaths. Imagine stepping out of your body and turning to take a good look at yourself from the outside. Are you relaxed or do you look stressed, tired or ill at ease? Take a closer look. How does your face look? Is your jaw tense and tight? Are you frowning or is your forehead smooth? How is your posture? Does your head jut forward constantly? Is your body tense and tight – look at your shoulders, and are your fists clenched? Do you constantly need to cross your legs? Do you look relaxed? Now step back inside yourself and explore how you feel on the inside. Do you feel anxious? If so, do you know why you are anxious? Is your mind cluttered with worrying thoughts? Or you are you at ease with yourself and the world around you?

around 75 per cent of the benefits that sleep brings. Proper relaxation training aims to calm the emotions and still the mind as well as the physical body.

Relaxation is a skill that needs to be learned just like any other. To relax means making a conscious decision to let go, to enter your inner world. Once there you can work through any challenges you may face and focus on your goals and your means of achieving them.

In the same way that you made a committed decision to get fit, you now need to do the same with the mental preparation that will enable you to achieve your fitness goals. The optimum state in which to think yourself fit is a relaxed one.

Environment

The first step is to make sure your environment is a relaxing one. It needs to be warm because the body becomes cooler as your muscles relax. It is important to ensure that you choose a time when you are unlikely to be disturbed, and be sure to disconnect the telephone. The best time to relax is normally first thing in the morning or last thing at night, when the mind is more likely to be in a state naturally conducive to relaxation.

The three most comfortable supported positions in which to relax are lying down, sitting with your back against a chair and sitting in a chair using cushions to lean forward on a table. Make sure that your legs are uncrossed and your arms are in a comfortable position, and, if you are sitting, that your feet are on the floor. I'm now going to introduce you to three different relaxation techniques. You may, if you wish, use a partner to read the instructions out to you. Alternatively, read the instructions onto a tape that you can play them back to yourself again and again.

Reciprocal Relaxation

This method works by instructing the body to reverse what would be its usual reaction to stress.

Get into a comfortable position in which you can completely relax. Focus on your breathing for a few moments: inhale through the nose and exhale out through the mouth. Spend some time just following your breathing and telling yourself that 'My mind is now completely relaxed.' As you inhale, breathe in stillness and relaxation; as you exhale, breathe out all the clutter in your mind. Now you're ready to turn your attention to your whole body, working your way down from your shoulders to your feet.

SHOULDERS: Spend a few moments pulling your shoulders down towards your feet – then release. Feel your shoulders relax and sit comfortably.

ELBOWS: Without lifting arms, move your elbows so that they are out and open. Pause to experience the feeling of your arms turned away from their sides, elbows resting gently on the floor, table or chair.

HANDS: Keeping the heel of your hand on the support (floor or bed) extend your fingers. Stop stretching and feel the heel of your hand resting on the support, your fingers separated and 'long'.

WHOLE BODY: Push your whole body into the support. Stop pushing and feel your whole body relaxed and your weight supported by the floor, chair or table.

LEGS: Push your feet away from your face with your toes pointed. Stop pushing and feel your legs and feet loosen so they are relaxed and heavy. Adjust your knees until they are comfortable.

HIPS: Turn your hips outwards. Stop turning and feel your feet and knees turn out and the muscles in your lower body loosen and become heavy.

FACE: Close your eyes and, with your mouth closed too, focus on dragging your tongue and jaw down. Stop and feel the jaw get heavy and your tongue lying in the middle of your mouth. Smooth your forehead up into your hair and through to the back of your skull. Stop and feel your skin and facial muscles relax and smooth.

HEAD: Feel the support (floor or bed) supporting your head. Now just feel waves of relaxation flow from the top of your head to the tips of your toes.

Progressive Relaxation

This involves tensing then relaxing muscle groups, which will promote your awareness of the difference between physical tension and relaxation. You may want to play some gentle relaxing music while you do this exercise. As before, get yourself into a comfortable position. Focus your attention on your breathing. Tell yourself that every time you breathe out you will relax a little more by breathing away all the tightness in your body.

FEET: Tighten the muscles in your feet. Feel your toes curling. Hold this tension for a count of four and then let go. Say to yourself, 'My feet are relaxing now.'

CALVES AND THIGHS: Tighten the muscles in your calves and thighs, back, front, inner and outer. Hold for a count of four – then let go. See the muscles in your calves and thighs completely loosen and say to yourself, 'My legs are relaxing now.'

BUTTOCKS, LOWER BACK AND ABDOMEN: Tighten your buttocks and abdominal muscles. Feel these muscles tightening and hold for a count of four. As you let go, be aware of all the tension leaving these muscles as they completely relax.

CHEST AND BACK: Direct your attention now to your chest and back muscles: tighten them and hold for a count of four – then just allow your chest and back muscles to completely relax. In your mind, see how your chest and back muscles expand as you breathe in and fall as you breathe out.

ARMS: Tighten the muscles in your upper arms, lower arms, elbows, wrists and finally your fists – hold for a count of four. Now allow your arms to relax and hang loosely by your side supported by the floor, chair or table.

SHOULDERS: Hunch up your shoulders and tighten the muscles in your neck. Hold for a count of four. Now let go completely and allow your shoulders to settle in a comfortable position free of all tension. Your neck should feel 'long'.

HEAD AND FACE: Tighten all the muscles in your head and face. Tighten your scalp muscles and make a face. Scrunch up your forehead, your mouth, your eyes – even scrunch up your ears if you can. Hold for a count of four. And now relax and let go completely.

Feel waves of relaxation flowing from the top of your head to the tips of your toes.

Physiological Relaxation

The aim of physiological relaxation is to relax all the muscles and organs of the body. It also uses visualization to promote mental relaxation. The following is a relaxation 'script' to record and play back to yourself.

'Get into a comfortable position in which you can completely relax. Close your eyes and focus your attention on your breathing. Take three deep breaths. Inhale through the nose and fill out your ribs and abdomen. Now exhale through the mouth. [Pause.] As you breathe be aware of your lungs filling every nerve, muscle, cell in your body with life-giving oxygen. Feel your ribs and abdomen lift as you breathe in and fall as you breathe out, lift as you breathe in and fall as you breathe out. Just be aware of the sensations in your body as you focus your attention on your breathing. [Pause.] Now, as you breathe evenly, rhythmically and naturally, be aware of all the muscles in your body, from the top of your head to the tips of your toes. Bring your attention to your feet and relax the muscles there. [Pause.] Now feel that relaxation spreading to the muscles in and around your ankles and calves, both front and back. [Pause.] As you begin to feel waves of relaxation flow to your lower limbs, allow your awareness to spread to your thighs – front, back, outer and inner – and hips and all the muscles surrounding them. Relax these muscles now. [Pause.] As you relax all the muscles in your lower body spend a few moments breathing even more relaxation into them. [Pause.] Feel those waves of relaxation flowing to the upper body, starting with the lower, middle and upper back. Be aware of the back muscles expanding and falling with every breath you take. [Pause.] Spend some time enjoying the rhythm of your breathing as you now focus on your abdominal muscles. See those muscles as a corset holding in your internal organs. See your internal organs slowing down and working at a natural pace. See them working at their natural rhythm now. [Pause.] See the relaxation flowing now to the muscles in your chest. Be aware of both your chest and abdominal muscles rising as you breathe in and falling as you breathe out, rising as you breathe in and falling as you breathe out. As the muscles in the lower and upper limbs begin to feel heavy and relaxed, allow the muscles in your shoulders to relax as well, releasing all the tension there. [Pause.] And now feel those waves spreading to the upper and lower arms, wrists, hands, fingers and fingertips. Feel your arms get loose and limp and supported by the floor, chair or table. [Pause.] Now see your neck muscles relax and the muscles in your face become smoother and smoother with every breath you take. Relax the muscles around your chin, jaw, forehead and eyes. See those muscles become smoother and smoother. [Pause.] Feel the waves of relaxation flowing from the top your head to the tips of your toes.'

When you want to experience these feelings of relaxation again just say 'Relax your body now.' Those words will immediately take you back.

Deepening Your Relaxation

After physical relaxation, you may further relax your mind by using the following 'deepeners'.

SEE YOURSELF: at the top of a flight of steps. There are 15 in total. Start to take one step at a time and with every step you take you double your relaxation. Fifteen: you feel more relaxed still. Fourteen: your mind is becoming relaxed. Thirteen: even more deeply relaxed. Twelve: your limbs feel heavier and heavier. Eleven: even more deeply relaxed still. Ten: body and mind relaxing even more. Nine: with every breath you take you go deeper. Eight: you are closing in on complete relaxation. Seven: your mind is feeling relaxed and still. Six: your limbs are getting heavier and heavier. Five: you're letting go now. Four: with every step you take you feel even more at ease. Three: closer still. Two: mind and body on the verge of complete relaxation. One: you are now completely relaxed.

IMAGINE A RULER: Its job is to measure your level of relaxation. It is numbered one to fifteen. What number on the ruler are you at now? Do you want to stay at that number or do you want to go deeper? If you want to go deeper just take three deep breaths, and on the third breath you will be at your desired level of relaxation. With each breath you become more and more relaxed.

*Do
one of the three relaxation and one of
the deepening exercises and then simply spend
some time in the most perfect imaginary place you can
think of. Associate into this place and see what you
see, hear what you hear and feel what you feel
– a sense of peace and tranquillity.*

COUNT BACKWARDS FROM 200: As you count backwards say 'deeper and deeper' between each number. So '200, deeper and deeper, 199, deeper and deeper' and so on. Keep on counting and as you count imagine the numbers getting smaller and smaller. The more you count the smaller the numbers become until the numbers literally disappear. When the numbers have disappeared you will be more relaxed than ever before.

The next step is to imagine the ideal environment in which to do your mental exercises. Think of your perfect setting: it might be a sandy beach, a landscape garden, or a tropical forest. It must be a place in which you feel safe and at ease.

Visualization

Perhaps one of the strongest mental tools that you can use to ensure success in exercise is to see your goal in your mind's eye. When you visualize something you are consciously taking control of your mind to create pictures that you want to manifest, to make true. Research has proven the power of this technique.

Top athletes use visualization to achieve peak performance. It is well known that Sally Gunnell prepared for her events with mental rehearsal. She would visualize every detail of an event for months beforehand as well as what would happen in the event itself. Linford Christie is another

Choose one of the three relaxation exercises then deepen your relaxation and visualize your positive place. Imagine that you are in a cinema. An image of you as you wish to be appears on the giant movie screen. Make the picture as perfect as you can by adding colour, clarity, confidence, a smile. Whatever is needed. Now just imagine that you are stepping into the picture and fully associating into the ideal you. How does it feel? Do you feel happy with yourself, confident? What do you see – a fitter, stronger you looking just the way that you want? What do you hear from yourself and the world around you? Now step out of the picture and blank the screen.

Now another image begins to emerge. See yourself working through your chosen exercise activities to reach your goal. See yourself turn up at the gym, get changed and perform your exercise in fine detail. See yourself working out with a positive attitude and perfect posture and technique. See yourself pacing your exercise so that you do the required amount of activity in a challenging but comfortable way. Hear yourself coaching yourself into position, giving yourself positive words of encouragement. Imagine how you will feel: pleased with yourself for your achievements, enjoying what you are doing and looking forward to feeling even better at the end of your session.

Now step into the movie of that experience. Associate into the picture and follow the instructions again, but this time see what you see, hear what you hear and feel what you feel. When you have fully associated into the experience, step out of the movie screen and bring those positive feelings with you. Every time you think of exercise in the future you say the words 'Fit and strong' to recapture this picture and those feelings.

How do you organize time in your mind? Think about something that happened a month, six months, a year ago. Physically point in the direction that it seems to come from. Now think of something you desire or expect to happen one month, six months, a year into the future. Point in the direction it seems to come from.

Now imagine a line of time that connects your past to your future. This is your timeline.

athlete who used visualization before and at the start of a race. But visualization is not only for athletes. Studies have been carried out to compare people who were sedentary and had never exercised before with others who were sedentary but visualized working out with heavy weights. The result was a measurable physiological trace of the second group's efforts. Imagining working out with weights sent messages along the brain's neural pathways to the muscles and thus created new neural patterns. Imagined activity activates the same neural pathways as real activity – the inner mind cannot tell the difference. However, that's not to say that you should just sit back and imagine yourself exercising – you still need to fully activate those muscles by doing the work.

Your Timeline

One very powerful technique in which visualization is used is timeline therapy. We all represent time in different ways. Often we litter our internal and external speech with expressions such as 'I can't see a future', 'I am focusing on the here and now' and 'He's living in the past.' We use language to code our experience of time and we organize that experience in a linear way.

Your timeline can be a very useful tool. You can use it to explore your behaviour in the past and present and to plan your future goals. The timeline exercises are a means of actualizing your goal by locating it at a definite place in the future. By taking control of time you can accelerate the process of reaching your goals; and you can pace yourself to get there by testing how you feel. You can create your future. You either act out your timeline physically or imagine it in your mind. The exercise on the opposite page is an adaptation of one devised by Jeffrey Hodges in his book *Sportsmind*. By putting mind to muscle, you can use visualization for greater gains from physical exercise. You can use visualization for better

Imagine
a line of time that represents your future.
Give the line a colour and see how long or short it is. Is it
straight or curvy? Does it branch off in different directions? Now
take your exercise goal and walk into the future to a time when you will
realistically have achieved it. You may want to try a few different places to find
the one that feels right. Put a frame around this goal. Leave this picture of your
goal in the future and travel back to the present. As you look into the future
become aware of the journey that it will to achieve your goal. Travel into the
future and place markers along the way as reference points so that you can
measure your progress. Think about what you need to be seeing,
hearing and feeling at those
markers.

Now
step into your goal picture and associate
with those powerful feelings and what it is like to be
strong, fit and healthy. Spend a few moments fully absorbing these
feelings. Step back on to the timeline and travel back towards the
present bringing these feelings with you. When you get back to the present
create a trigger phrase such as 'strong and fit'. You can use this trigger phrase
to bring on these powerful
positive feelings at any
time in the
future.

As
you now step into your goal picture, be
aware of what it feels like to be strong and fit and
healthy. Fully associate into those powerful feelings. Then as you
step back on to your timeline to travel back to the present bring these
feelings with you by walking backwards and focusing on that main goal
picture; pick up all those great feelings of success at each marker point.
When you get back to the present, create a trigger phrase, such as
'strong and fit and healthy', that you can use at any time
in the future to bring on these positive
feelings.

Stand

or sit with your arms down by your sides and make fists with your hands. Imagine holding a 5-10kg dumbbell. Keeping your elbows by your sides, imagine the extra resistance as you bring your hand towards your shoulders and 'curl' your biceps for a count of two. See the tension in your muscles as they lift the imagined weight. Now feel the tension as you curl up. Slowly lower your arm for a count of four

body awareness, to increase flexibility and to monitor the intensity of your exercise, to make your exercise more effective and to push yourself to do those extra repetitions.

So often we limit ourselves in life by thinking we can do only so much. If we look beyond our limiting beliefs there are so many possibilities. Think of all the things that the human race is capable of. We get faster and stronger and break all kinds of records year in, year out. Think of Roger Banister making the decision to run a mile in less than four minutes when no one believed it was possible. He did it, and now the best athletes can't imagine completing the mile in more than four minutes.

How does this apply to you? Can you do more than you think?

You'll

need a towel to do this stretch. Lie on your back with your right leg bent and your left leg straight. Hook the towel behind the ankle of your left leg. Keeping your buttocks on the floor, gently ease your straight leg as far as you comfortably can towards your chest. Hold the position and feel the stretch on the back of the thigh. Now visualize yourself gently taking the stretch a little further than you think you can. Make sure you keep your body in the correct posture – buttocks on the floor. Ensure that you don't jerk or bounce. Gently ease yourself into the position and hold that stretch for ten seconds.

Changing the Negative Self-talk

What about the internal dialogue that might have caused havoc in your life up till now? You may believe that it is difficult to change the habits of a lifetime and suddenly start thinking positively about exercise or fitness. But the fact is you weren't born thinking negatively. You have learned to do so in the same way that you have learned any skill – to walk, talk, brush your teeth, ride a bike. If this is a skill that you have learned then you unlearn it if you choose. How? By developing new positive language patterns that will empower you to achieve your exercise and life goals. You develop positive language by changing the words that you use from negative to positive. You then repeat those words over and over again until they become true in your mind. When the words become true you will find that you begin to think differently and move towards your goals. Where exercise and fitness are concerned, this means that you can act as your own personal trainer. You can talk yourself into doing exercise, you can motivate and encourage yourself, raise your self-confidence, teach yourself exercise skills and push yourself when you need to be challenged physically.

You may now realize that awareness is the first step on the way to taking control of your thought processes. And after awareness comes action – you need to consciously challenge yourself and the thought that you have just had. You need to do this by giving yourself a word to stop you in your tracks. I use the word 'halt'. It is important to ensure that you do not beat yourself up with another statement that will compound your original negative talk. I found myself doing this in the past. I would have a negative thought then call myself a 'dummy' for having had that thought. And how negative is that? Whenever I catch myself having a negative thought now I listen to it and I simply smile or laugh. I may also change the tone by using a silly voice. That seems to break the cycle.

By first intervening when you have a negative thought you ready yourself to make it a positive statement instead. It is best to have a statement that coincides with the beliefs and values that empower you and are in keeping with your identity. If you choose a statement that you just do not believe, no matter how hard you try, it won't work. But if you have difficulty in believing but you still want to believe, say the word or affirmation anyway. It is normal and natural to start off with resistance so it is important to persevere. Once you whole-heartedly believe something you will be living it.

Affirmations

Affirmations are positive statements that will empower you to reach your fitness goals (I have given some examples on page 117). You can repeat your affirmations while you are doing your relaxation exercises. You can write them down and stick them somewhere where you will see them – on a mirror or a fridge door or on your office desk. You can say them out loud or quietly to yourself. You can even sing and draw them – just find as many different ways as you can to repeat them.

- You may want to develop some sort of routine to ensure you have space in your mind to think, say and write your affirmations. For example, setting time aside for ten minutes in the morning and at night.
- Begin by repeating your fitness affirmations twice a day for a few minutes in the morning and then in the evening. Build up to five minutes in the morning and in the evening before going to bed.
- Ensure that your affirmations will help you reach your goal.
- Put all pressing problems in the past tense.
- Make sure your statements are to the point and easy to remember.
- You can devise affirmations for small, medium and large goals.
- Focus your attention on your goal as you repeat your affirmation.
- Give yourself no more than two affirmations to work on at a time.
- Find different ways to make your affirmations.
- Repeat your affirmations with feeling and meaning as if they are true – what the mind believes becomes truth. Act as if your affirmations were true.
- Persevere! It takes 21 days to create a habit. You may see changes earlier but you then need to practise, practise, practise!

Your mind will do what you programme it to do. When your mind is deeply relaxed it lacks critical awareness and is very literal in its interpretations.

The following principles are guidelines to follow to ensure that your affirmations will be accepted in a positive way by your subconscious mind. **BE POSITIVE:** focus on achievement when you make up your affirmations. You need to highlight the benefits to be enjoyed and the positive good that will come from achieving your goals. Make sure you are focusing on what you do want and not on what you don't want. Ensure that you use positive language. For example, change 'I must try to get to the gym' to 'I get to the gym every day', and 'I am no longer bored with exercise' to 'I look forward to exercising.'

Be specific. Be realistic. Be active. Be repetitive. Be in the present!

BE SPECIFIC: in the same way that you should be really specific about the goals that you want to achieve, you must also devise affirmations that are tailored to them. Choose words that target your goal clearly and precisely. For example, if you want to tone up, 'I am getting fitter every day' could become 'My muscles are becoming stronger and more toned every day.'

BE REALISTIC: an essential part of setting any goal is being realistic about your achievements. If you give yourself a goal that is too much of a challenge you are likely to give up. For example, 'I make sure I exercise every day to lose two stones in weight' sounds very ambitious if, like many, you have a busy life and find it difficult to exercise three times a week. And 'two stones' can be an imposing figure. Try instead, 'As I exercise consistently three times a week I get closer and closer to achieving my goal weight.'

BE ACTIVE: bring your thoughts to life! They may look like a bunch of words on a page, but you can make what you will of them. Use descriptive 'action' words to make you want to jump out of your chair and get going. 'I like exercise' could become 'I really enjoy exercise', ' I look forward to exercising ', 'I love exercise', 'I am supremely confident about reaching my goals.'

BE REPETITIVE: when you repeat an affirmation and give it your attention the more you strengthen the suggestion and the more likely it is to become true. You can repeat the same affirmation over and over again. Alternatively you can find different ways to say the same thing: 'Fitness is easy for me', 'I really enjoy the process of getting fit', 'I look forward to my gym sessions', 'I have a strong desire to work my body.'

BE IN THE PRESENT: you need to focus on your goals as if you were already accomplishing them. So it will be confusing if you say 'I exercise better than I did last week ', because you will have already experienced exercising last week. If your point of focus was on last week's exercise then you are more likely to emulate last week's workout. The subconscious mind responds quite literally to specific commands.

The following is a list of affirmations to use in conjunction with all of these principles. Do make up your own as well.

- 'I always remember to make time in my diary for exercise.'
- 'My heart is strong and healthy.'
- 'It is easy for me to exercise four times a week.'
- 'My muscles are becoming more toned now.'
- 'My muscles are strong and powerful.'
- 'I am growing stronger every day.'
- 'I love my body shape.'
- 'My body is strong and sexy.'
- 'I accept the shape that I was born with.'
- 'As I exercise I have more energy and vitality.'
- 'I look forward to exercising.'
- 'I exercise regularly and consistently.'
- 'I look forward to reaching my ideal weight in three months' time.'
- 'I enjoy exercise.'
- 'It is easy to find the time for exercise.'
- 'I am now getting closer and closer to my fitness goals.'
- 'I am confident that I am reaching my exercise goals.'
- 'My confidence grows every day.'
- 'There is enough time for me to exercise and I make time for exercise.'

You can enhance and reinforce your desire to get fit by building in positive affirmations to your visualization

The following are useful exercise 'scripts'. Rewrite them, expand them and make them specific to your needs. Remember, if you are memorizing the words use the first-person 'I' and if you are transferring them to a tape use the second-person 'you'. (I've used the first person in my examples.)

TIME: 'Now that I have made the decision to achieve my fitness goals, it is easy to find time for fitness. I make time to exercise regularly. I exercise three times a week and I enjoy the thought of exercise. I look forward to planning my diary and I make exercise appointments every week. I make good use of the 45 minutes that I spend at the gym. I focus on my muscles when I exercise and I know that I am working my body efficiently and effectively.'

SELF-IMAGE: 'I know that the first step on the way to achieving my ideal body weight is to accept the shape that I was born with. I accept the shape I was born with and I know that I can be the best that I can be within that body shape. I know and understand that I am wonderful in my own unique way. I will find ways to achieve the best body shape that I can.'

Imagine
you are in your perfect place or in that
cinema in your mind. Create an image of you as you wish
to be. Your body looks strong and fit. You are full of health
and vitality. Step into the picture and just listen to that new positive
dialogue: 'My muscles are becoming stronger and stronger every day',
'My posture is upright and purposeful', 'I feel full of energy and
vitality'. Be aware of what it feels like to have strong muscles
and a perfect posture, what it feels like to be full of
energy, vitality and confidence.

MOTIVATION: 'I act through my body to achieve my goals. Therefore I know a strong, fit body will serve me well in every area of my life. I know that it is never too late to start exercising and I enjoy the thought of exercise. I have a strong desire to get fit and now I look forward to exercise knowing that I will soon see the results that I desire in my body and mind. I enjoy fitness challenges. Every step I take is moving me towards my fitness goals. Fitness is easy for me. I enjoy the process of getting fit. I stick to my fitness routine every day.'

CONSISTENCY: 'I'm becoming fitter and fitter every day and I am consistent in my efforts to achieve my exercise goals. I know that I am establishing healthy lifestyle patterns for life. I exercise regularly and I am now happy and confident that these patterns are here to stay. I continue to have a strong desire to get fit. I have fun with fitness and I always remember to fit exercise into my diary.'

CONFIDENCE: 'I am becoming more and more confident as every day goes by. And I look forward to achieving my exercise goals. My confidence increases every day as I acknowledge my achievements. I acknowledge my success. I recognize all my talents and special qualities, and my abilities grow and grow every day as I become fitter and more skilful. Every time I reach a goal I give myself praise. I enjoy my success.'

Finally, you can enhance and reinforce your desire to get fit by building in positive affirmations to your visualization exercises.

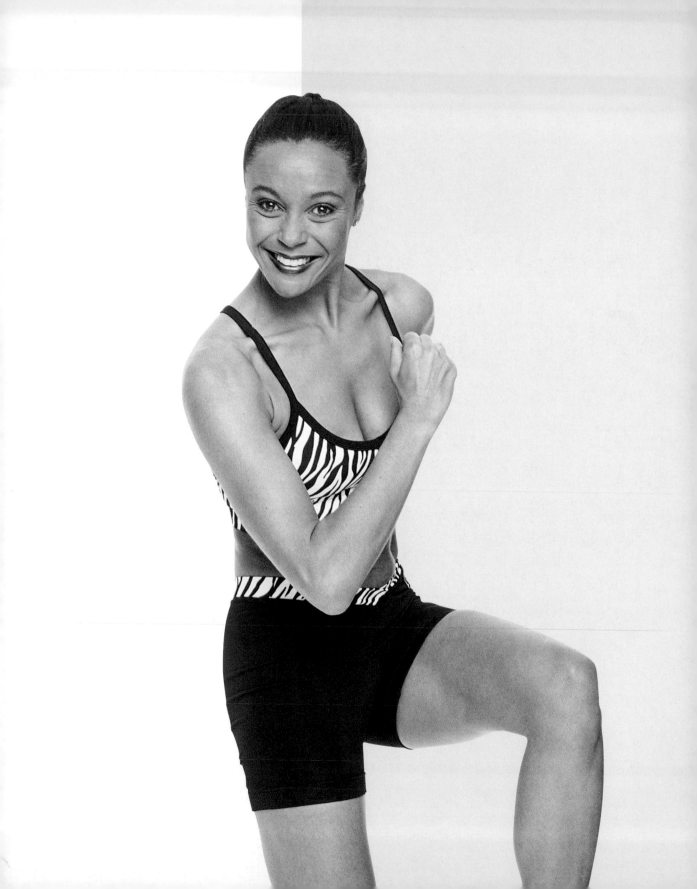

Chapter 7

The Fitness Circuit

So, what further tools will enable you to reach your fitness goals?

Flick back to the logical levels of fitness and re-read the capability

section. You may recall that when you learn a new skill that you go

through a number of competence levels before you automatically

become skilful at a given task. A further mind tool that will help

with the transition of competence levels is patience and the ability

to learn and workout at a pace that suits you.

The Think Yourself Fitness Circuit

When you pace yourself you are working at a speed that matches your skills and your ability. You can use your senses to help you with this. Remember to be aware of negative self-talk and consciously stop and replace any negative suggestions with positive ones. Pace yourself by using your auditory skills to talk yourself into a positive position and motivate yourself to keep going. You can remind yourself that each step of the way you are working towards your goals. You can use your visual skills to do the exercises in the following pictures then recreate them in your mind's eye so that you work out using good technique and posture. You can use visualization to enhance your performance, particularly in the strength and stretches sections. You can use your kinaesthetic skills to enhance your body awareness, to focus your mind on your muscles and to monitor the intensity of the exercises that you are doing. Be guided by how you feel. Lastly, remember it is your perception of fitness that can make it an uncomfortable experience so focus on the positive.

You will find that as you become better at the exercises you will be able to get into position faster so you really will be able to focus on the quality of your workout and get the best results.

The Three Ss

For a well-rounded exercise programme there are three principles to learn.

- **STRENGTH**
- **STAMINA**
- **SUPPLENESS**

Strength

When you perform strength training exercises you work individual groups of muscles by stimulating them to become stronger and larger. This helps you to build and maintain your muscle mass throughout your lifetime. But don't worry ladies, this does not mean that you will bulk up. Women have less muscle mass than men and considerably less testosterone. Strength training will give your muscles a more toned look. It will also help balance muscle groups and promote good posture. It will also help to fight off degenerative diseases such as osteoporosis. Strength training means working groups of muscles or individual muscles against resistance. That resistance can come in the form of body weight or you can use external resistance such as free weights, dynabands or gym equipment. You can make up your own resistance by filling plastic bottles with sand or using back packs.

SETS AND REPS

When you perform resistance work you use sets and reps (repititions) in order to progress and get the best results. Repetitions are the repeated movement of a weight to challenge your muscles and bring them to a point of fatigue. A set is a group of repetitions. Generally there are two sets to an exercise programme. To get results you need to exercise your muscles to a point where you cannot do any more. At this stage you may find that your muscles feel tired or depleted of energy. If you are a complete beginner you may need to build up on the amount of repetitions that you do. You may want to start with setting yourself the goal of ten reps and build up to twenty. You also want to make sure that you give yourself a day's break in between training the same muscle groups and do no more than three sessions a week on the same muscle group.

Stamina

If your goal is to tone your muscles and improve your posture then strength work is clearly for you. But if you want to lose excess pounds

Cardiovascular fitness encourages your heart and lungs to pump blood and supply oxygen to all your muscles and organs.

then you need to combine strength work with exercise that promotes stamina. In other words, you need to improve your staying power. Cardiovascular fitness encourages your heart and lungs to pump blood and supply oxygen to all the muscles and organs of your body. It is aerobic exercise that promotes cardiovascular fitness. Aerobic means 'with oxygen' and consists of continous movements performed over a period of time that use all the major muscle groups of the body. The British Heart Foundation suggests following the government recommendation for physical activity for adults of a minimum of 30 minutes of aerobic activity at moderate intensity (such as brisk walking, cycling or climbing the stairs) five or more days of the week.

Cardiovascular exercise can be done in many ways. Different sports such as tennis, football, rowing, running, cycling, walking, swimming, step, aerobics, slide, treadmill, rowing, spinning and dance all provide excellent aerobic exercise. It is recommended that you work out aerobically for 20 to 30 minutes to burn optimum calories and exercise your heart and lungs effectively and efficiently. So you need to make sure that you can find activities that will allow you do this. If you are a complete beginner you may want to build from 10 mins up to 20 then up to 30.

Suppleness

When you have a supple body your joints are able to move freely through their full range of motion and your muscles are able to stretch easily to their maximum length. In today's society life itself can affect your suppleness. The tensions, stresses and strains of every day life can affect your muscles, causing them to be tight and tense. As a result, your posture can also be affected and imbalances in muscle groups can occur. For example, if you sit over a computer for long periods of time your back muscles may become weak and overstretched and your chest muscles may tighten so that you develop round shoulders. Other common postural problems include short hamstrings, slack buttock muscles, tight hip flexors and weak abdominal musclesl. If you don't move your body you will lose your innate ability to move freely. The aim of stretching as part of exercise is to maintain and develop suppleness by increasing your range of movement through various movements. Stretching promotes better posture and relaxes and reduces muscle tension and enables your body to move more freely and efficiently. At the end of an exercise session you need to stretch to alleviate the tightness in your muscles caused by the shortening contractions produced by exercise. The safest and most common method of stretching during exercise is static stretching. This is a slow gradual stretch in a held position.

Stretching promotes better posture, relaxes and reduces muscle tension.

The Fitness Circuit

The following workout is designed for both beginner and intermediate levels of fitness. It is the perfect combination of a strength training circuit to tone your muscles and aerobic moves that can burn excess calories. With the strength section, make sure you build up to 20 reps and when that becomes easy, increase your resistance by using more weight. Use the warm up moves and make them aerobic by exaggerating them to make them bigger and wider. Put more energy into them. You can incorporate these moves into your circuit for cardiovascular fitness and to burn up excess calories. Incorporate the aerobic moves in-between each strength move. At the end of the fitness circuit it is essential that you do your cool down stretches to bring your muscles back into balance and to develop flexibility and alleviate the tightness that can occur. Make sure you hold each of the stretches for 15 to 30 seconds. Always consult your doctor before beginning a new exercise programme, especially if you have any medical conditions that may affect your ability to participate in exercise.

Warm up

Before you start exercising you need to prepare your body by warming up properly. This is an essential part of the session so DO NOT SKIP IT. You warm up to prepare your muscles for exercise by increasing the blood flow to the muscles, gradually raising your body temperature and loosening your joints. This makes them less vulnerable to injury. A good warm up also promotes good body awareness and prepares your mind to focus on the exercise ahead. Whilst moving your body ensure that you maintain a neutral spine position throughout. You do this by tightening your abdominals to ensure you do not over-arch your back. Do the following moves until your body feels warm and your muscles are pliable. Notice how great you feel as you find your body loosening up.

Enviroment

You need to have a clear area with enough space to gently jog or briskly march around the room or the garden. Take around seven minutes to fully warm up. Use some motivating and stimulating music if you wish, with beats around 128 to 130 per minute. Spend around 20 seconds with each move.

1 Begin by marching on the spot or around the room. Make sure as you march you do so lightly. No stomping – walk through your feet from heel to toe and swing your arms naturally. March up and down, forwards and backwards – in fact just march anywhere you like.
2 Now step on to the right foot and kick your heels behind you. Gradually lift your heels higher and higher as if to kick your bottom. Alternate between each leg. Make sure that as you kick your abdominals remain tight throughout and your spine remains neutral.
3 Go back to a march.

4 Now step on to your right foot keeping your right knee slightly soft and raise your left knee in front of you up to hip level. Bring your opposite elbow to your knee. Keep your upper body relaxed. Alternate between each leg.
5 Go back to a march.

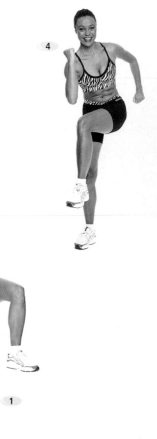

6 Change your march into a skip. If you have forgotten how, just imagine you are back at school, skipping in the school playground.
7 Go back to a march.

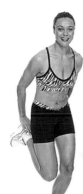

8 Now jog gently on the spot making sure you pick your feet up off the ground. Put your hands on your bottom with palms facing away from you. Aim for your heels to hit your hands.
9 Go back to a march.

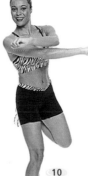

10 Repeat the back to heel kicks (8) but this time bring your arms out in front of you across your chest.
11 Go back to a march.

12 Stand on your left leg and bring your right leg forward to a point and tap it in front of you. Your arms are by your side with your hands pressing behind you. Alternate between each leg.
13 Go back to a march.

A good warm up promotes body awareness and prepares the mind to focus on the exercise ahead.

16 Back to position 4 but this time punch arms up towards the ceiling.

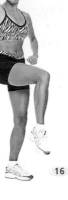

14 Stand on your left leg and bring your right leg forward but this time flex your foot in front of you. Raise your arms up to shoulder level and then let them fall. Alternate between each leg.
15 Go back to a march.

To Mobilise Your Joints

2 SPINE: Stand with feet hip distance apart and knees bent. Lean forward, placing your hands on your thighs. Keep your spine in a neutral position by tightening your abdominals. Now, keeping your shoulders relaxed, tuck your pelvis right under and lift up through the spine by rounding your back to make a bridge. Keep looking at the floor. Now, press your hips back out behind you and return to the starting position remembering to maintain that neutral spine.

1 WAIST: Stand with feet hip distance apart and knees slightly soft. Keeping your hips facing forward, place your hands on your shoulders and rotate your torso to the right for 20 seconds. Return to the front and then turn to the left for 20 seconds. Return to the start position.

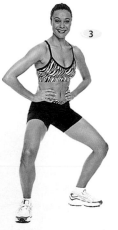

Just acknowledge how great you feel as you find your body loosening up.

3 KNEE BENDS: Stand with feet shoulder width apart. Turn your toes out to ten to and ten past the hour of a clock. Put your hands on your hips. Bend your knees out over your toes. As you straighten your legs ensure that your knees remain soft.

5 NECK ROLLS: Stand with feet hip distance apart and knees soft, maintaining that neutral spine. Gently rotate your head so that your chin comes over towards your right shoulder, then down towards your chest, then over to your left shoulder.

4 SHOULDER CIRCLES: Stand with feet hip distance apart and knees soft but not bent. Maintain a neutral spine. Take your hands to your shoulders and circle them forwards, up, back and down. Make sure your movements are smooth and controlled.

The Circuit

Now your muscles are warm it is time to focus on conditioning your body. Remember, although the workout is primarily a strength circuit, you can add your aerobic moves to it. Use the moves that you have learnt from the warm up but make them bigger and wider and more intense so you can also use the following exercises to work your heart and burn those calories.

Step up and down on your stairs, beginners start with the first step, intermediates the second or third step. Make sure you place your whole foot on the stair and that you step lightly. As you come off the stair, step through the ball of the foot on to the heel. *No stomping*. Use a skipping rope and skip. Make sure both knees are soft when you land and work through from the back of the foot to the heel. Work at a pace that is comfortable. Do each of these for 30 to 45 seconds depending on whether you are a beginner or more advanced. Make sure you pace yourself. Work at a level that challenges you but is safe and effective. Monitor the intensity of your workout using the talk test. If you can talk easily you are not working hard enough. If you are huffing and puffing and cannot hold a conversation at all, you are working too hard. You need to be able to hold a breathy conversation.

For the strength circuit, it is important that the exercises challenge your muscles. If you find that after 30 seconds you are not challenged, do 45 seconds instead. When the exercises become easy you need to find some form of resistance that will fatigue your muscles in this time.

Calf Raises

BEGINNERS

Stand with feet hip distance apart and knees slightly soft. If you wish you may use a support.

ACTION

- Raise your heels off the ground for two counts, pushing into the balls of your feet then slowly lower for two counts.
- Focus on your big and middle toes, not on the outside of your foot.
- Make sure your upper body remains upright and avoid arching your back by tightening your abdominals.

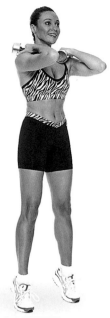

ADVANCED

Add some dumbbells. Either hold them by your sides or on your shoulders.

Chair Squat

BEGINNERS

Stand in front of a chair with a seat no lower than your knee line and with your feet shoulder width apart and your toes facing forwards. Place your hands on your thighs

ACTION

- Lean forwards pulling in your abdominal muscles and pressing your hips out behind you as if to sit in the chair, for two counts.
- Allow your buttocks to touch the seat of the chair before pushing up through your heels and standing up again for four counts, squeezing your buttocks as you do so.

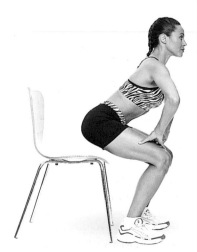

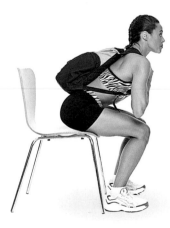

INTERMEDIATE

Now do the same with a backpack that has evenly distributed weight in it, ideally with the weight placed on the upper part of the back. Start with a few books weighing a total of 5lbs and then add more. As you get stronger it is essential that you maintain a good posture and that you do not allow your back to over arch.

Inner Thigh Squeeze

BEGINNERS

Stand with your bodyweight on your left leg. Tighten your abdominal muscles. Place your hands on your hips and extend your right leg to the side as far as it is comfortable.

ACTION

- Press your right foot forward into the floor and drag it back towards your left leg, squeezing your inner thigh and buttocks as you do so.

VARIATION AND ADVANCED

Lie on your side with both legs together. Raise yourself on to your elbows. Bring the top leg behind you and put your foot flat on the floor. Add a weight to this exercise to increase the intensity. The bottom leg remains straight. Press down on the inner thigh with a weight.

ACTION

- With your foot flexed, lift the lower leg so that you feel the muscles working in the inner thigh then gently lower it for two counts, keeping your heel off the ground.
- Make sure your knees and toes are facing forward and that you keep your foot off the ground as you come back to the starting position.

Outer Thigh

BEGINNERS

Stand by a chair for support. Very gently shift your weight on to your left leg and keep the knee soft (not bent or locked straight). Take your right leg out to the side, with your toes touching the floor.

ACTION

- Squeeze your buttocks, tighten your abdominals and lift your right leg for two counts squeezing into the outer thigh muscles as you do so. Make sure you lift from the hips as you raise your leg out to the side.
- Make sure your foot, knees and hips are facing forward.

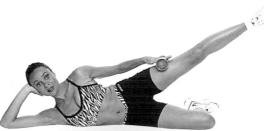

VARIATION AND ADVANCED

Lie on your side with legs straight and hips facing forward. Bend your elbow and rest your head on your hand. You can increase the intensity by using your hands to press down on the outer thigh or using a weight.

ACTION

- Raise the top leg for two counts and lower it for two counts. Make sure as you lift you keep your abdominals tight, and hips, knees and toes facing forward. Ensure that your hips stay forward throughout and do not roll back. Squeeze the outer thigh muscle as you lift.

Press Ups

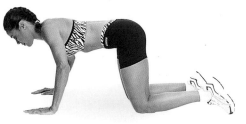

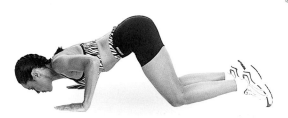

BEGINNERS

Kneel on all fours ensuring that your knees are protected. Your knees should be under your hips and your arms should be shoulder width apart and beneath your shoulders. Keep your back straight by pulling in your abdominal muscles.

ACTION

- Keeping your body weight over your arms, bend your elbows to bring your chest towards the floor. Keep your head in line with your body. Hold this position for two counts. Now press up to the starting position by straightening your arms. Ensure that your elbows remain soft as you do.

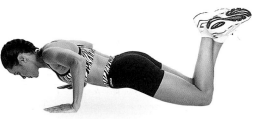

INTERMEDIATE

Do the same as above but take your knees further back as in the picture.

Full Length Press Up

Lie in a straight line flat on the ground, like a plank. Place your hands on the floor at shoulder width apart. Tuck your toes under and hold in your abdominals. Extend your arms and press up through the palms of your hands ensuring you do not lock your elbows.

ACTION

- Lean forward so your body weight is over your arms. Bend them for two counts, bringing your chest towards the floor and then press up to the starting position.
- Make sure your back is straight.
- Hold your abs in.
- Keep your elbows soft as you extend your arms.
- Keep your head in line with your body.

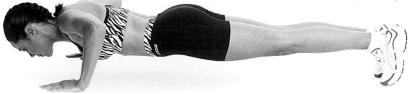

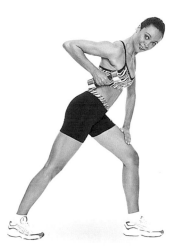

Single Arm Row

BEGINNERS

You need some added resistance for this
exercise so use a weight that will
allow you to do around 20 reps. If
you do not have weights take a
bottle of water and fill it with
sand and stones. Small ones for ladies, large ones for chaps.
Take a step forward with your left leg and bend it in front of
you. Your right leg should be straight behind you. Lean on your
left leg with your left arm and hold in your abdominal muscles.
Holding a weight in your right hand and facing the body, allow
the right arm to hang low towards the floor.

ACTION

- Pull the dumbbell towards your ribcage for two
  counts so that the elbow ends up at shoulder
  height, and then back for four counts. Make sure
  the elbow stays close to the waist as you lift.
- You can also use a chair or a bench or some other
  sturdy object to support yourself.
- Make sure you don't grip the weights too tightly.

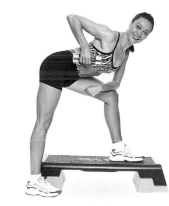

VARIATION

Use a step bench or chair.
Use a heavier weight for a more
advanced movement.

Bicep Curl

Sit or stand with your back in an upright posture. Hold in
your abdominal muscles and keep your chest lifted. Your
arms should hang by your sides with a weight in each hand.

ACTION

- Keeping your elbows and shoulders in a fixed position,
  curl the dumbbells towards your shoulders for two
  counts. Pause then lower for four counts
- Make sure your back is straight.
- Keep your elbows in.
- Keep your Shoulders fixed.

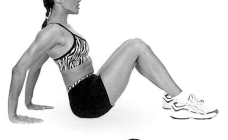

Triceps

BEGINNERS

Sit on the floor with your legs bent and your feet flat on the floor. Take your hands behind you. Make sure they are shoulder width apart with fingers facing forward.

ACTION

- Bend your elbows and lean back so that your body weight is on your arms. Hold in your abdominal muscles and make sure your hips and legs stay still. Press through the palm of the hand back into sitting position.

ADVANCED

You need a strong sturdy table, a sofa, the end of your bed or a step. Sitting on the edge of the step, place your hands behind you on the step, shoulder width apart and with your fingers facing forward. Hold the edge of the step and make sure your elbows face away from you.

ACTION

- Take your bodyweight off the step and bend your elbows to just below shoulder level taking your weight on to your arms. As you do this, bend your knees in line with your toes at a right angle. Lower your body down to the floor. Then straighten your arms without locking the elbows.
- Focus on keeping your bodyweight over your arms.
- Keep your back straight and close to the step.
- Keep your abdominal muscles in.
- Your movements should be slow and controlled.
- Avoid bouncing.
- Only lower yourself as far as is comfortable.
- Do the same as above but straighten your legs.

Back Extension

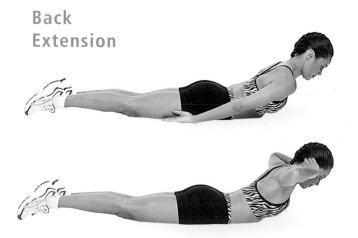

BEGINNERS

Lie on your front. You can either have your arms by your sides so your palms are on the floor or by your ears if you want a more advanced version.
Keep your hips and feet pressed to the floor and your face looking down at the floor.

ACTION

- Focus on using your lower back muscles to raise your chest and shoulders off the floor. Lift for two counts, hold two counts and lower for two counts.
- Only raise as far as is comfortable.
- Keep feet and hips pressed to the floor.
- Keep your head relaxed and in line with your body.

Abdominals

BEGINNERS

Lie on your back with your knees bent and your feet flat on the floor about hip distance apart. Ensure you have a neutral spine by tightening your abdominal muscles. Take your arms out in front of you.

ACTION

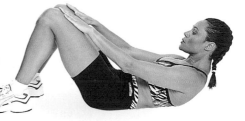

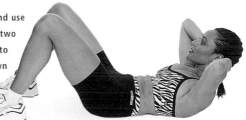

- Focus your mind on your abdominal muscles and use them to lift your shoulders off the ground for two counts, until they're at an angle of around 30 to 40 degrees from the ground. Slowly lower down for four counts.
- Aim to touch your knees.
- Let your abdominal muscles do the work.
- Relax your neck and let your head go.
- Make sure you are breathing normally and naturally.
- There should remain a gap between your chin and chest.

ADVANCED

Bend your elbows and place your fingers behind your head. Keep your elbows out and open as you use your abdominals to raise your shoulders off the ground.

Obliques

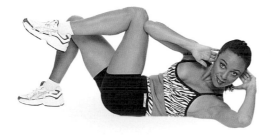

BEGINNERS

Lie on your back with your feet on the floor and your knees bent. Place one hand behind your ear and the other hand out on the floor for support.

ACTION

- Tighten your abdominal muscles and curl up and over diagonally for two counts, bringing your shoulder towards the opposite knee. Gently return to the starting position ensuring you keep your head off the ground as you do so.
- Repeat on the opposite side.

ADVANCED

Lie on your back with your knees bent and your feet slightly apart and flat on the floor. Bring your left ankle across your right knee and place your left arm to the side. Place your right hand behind your ear for support.

- Tighten your abdominals and bring your right shoulder towards your left knee for two counts and then back for two counts.
- Make sure your hips are firmly on the floor.
- Do not pull on your head.
- Keep your knee out to the side.

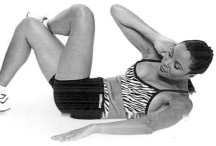

Well done for completing the circuit! Now it is time to cool down and stretch your muscles.

The Stretches

Well done for completing the circuit. Now it is time to cool down, stretch your muscles and develop your flexibility. Once you become accustomed to the different stretch positions you can use visualization to increase your flexibility. You do this by allowing your muscles to come to a point of tension then as the tension relaxes you visualize yourself stretching further. Remember your inner mind cannot tell the difference between the real and imaginary. As you see yourself in your mind's eyes so shall ye be! You then allow your body to follow that picture in your mind. Make sure you hold all stretches for at least 15 seconds and if you wish to increase your flexibility increase over a period of time up to one minute.

Put on some calming music and focus on relaxing.

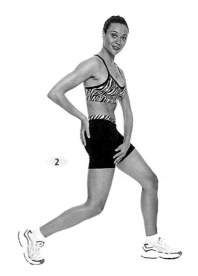

2 HIP FLEXOR STRETCH

You may need a wall or chair to help you balance. Stand with feet together. Take one leg behind you and lift the heel off the ground and keeping the ball of the foot on the ground. Bend your knees and tuck your pelvis right under. Make sure your feet are facing forward and keep your abdominals tight. Make sure your upper body is upright. Hold this position.

1 CALF STRETCH

You may need to use a support for balance.
Take a step forward with your left leg and bend the left knee. Make sure the right leg is straight with the heel pressed to the floor. Make sure the toes of both feet are facing forward and that a diagonal line runs from the heel of the back foot to the top of your head. Ensure your hips are facing forward. Hold the stretch for 15 seconds.
Now bring the right leg forward and bend your knee as if to sit back on the heel. Press the heel down and feel the stretch on the lower calf muscle. Make sure your body stays centred.

3 ABDUCTOR

Lie on your back with your knees bent and your feet together. Let your knees drop and press your inner thighs, pushing the souls of your feet together. Hold for 15 seconds. Breathe normally throughout.

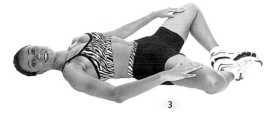

4 ABDUCTOR

Sitting in an upright position with both buttocks on the ground, stretch your legs out in front of you. Keeping the left leg extended, bend the right leg and bring it across the left leg at knee level.
Bring your left hand over your bent knee and place your right hand on the floor for support. Gently press your right knee in towards your body. Now stretch the other side. For a waist stretch turn your head and rotate your body to look directly over your shoulder.

Put on some calming music and focus on relaxing.

5 BUTT STRETCH

Lie on your back and bend your right knee towards you. Place your left foot on the floor with the knee bent. Take your right foot across your left knee. Bring your left knee up towards you with your hands at the back of the knee and hold. Then repeat with the other leg. Beginners, if you find this difficult you may want to keep your left foot flat on the floor and your right foot across your left knee. Sit up with your hands on the floor behind you for support.

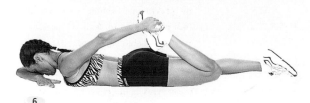

6 QUADRICEPS

Lie on your tummy with your hips pressed to the floor. Bend your left leg so that your heel is towards your buttocks. Take your left foot with your left hand and gently bring the heel closer to your buttocks tilting your pelvis as you do so. Make sure your body stays in a straight line. Now stretch the other side.

8 ABDOMINAL STRETCH

Lie on your tummy and place your hands on the floor in front of you at shoulder level, so that your elbows are in line with your shoulders. Push up on to your elbows by lifting your head and shoulders off the floor. Keep your hips, elbows and feet on the floor. Make sure your head stays in line with your body.

8

7 HAMSTRINGS

Lie on your back with your feet flat on the floor. Bend one leg and extend the other towards the ceiling. If you like you can use a towel and hook it around the extended leg. Gently bring the extended leg towards your chest until you feel a stretch in the back of the thigh. Hold for 15 seconds then change sides.

7

How do you feel? Remember this great feeling for the future.

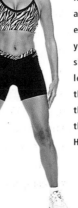

14 NECK STRETCH

In standing position with your feet apart and knees slightly soft, drop your right ear towards your right shoulder. Bring your right arm over your right shoulder to the left ear. Press the left shoulder towards the floor. You can do this by flexing your hand and pushing through the palm then relaxing it. Feel the stretch on the left side of the neck. Hold for 15 seconds then change sides.

9

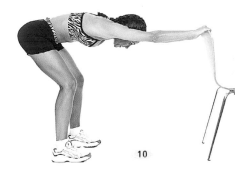

11 BACK STRETCH

Stand about two feet away from the arm of your chair or sofa with your body facing it. Lean forward, placing your hands on the inside of the armrest. Now bend your knees and press your hips out behind you as if you are about to sit down. Keep your head in line with your spine and make sure you don't bend your knees more than 90 degrees. Hold.

10

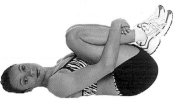

11

12 LOWER BACK STRETCH

Lie on your back and hug your knees towards your chest.

12

13 TRICEPS

Sit or stand maintaining an upright posture. Take your right arm over your head and bend the elbow. Bring the right hand to the left to support it just below the elbow. You can make this stretch more advanced by reaching your left arm up your back towards your right hand and holding onto your fingers of your right hand. Hold that stretch.

Well done! You have completed your fitness circuit! Did you use all your mental tools to get the most out of your performance? Did you acknowledge where you are in terms of levels of competence and know that you if you keep practising you will get to the next level soon? What about your pain and pleasure barriers? What was your perception of the effort and the physical sensations you felt? Were you able to tolerate those sensations of exercise? Did you use positive internal dialogue and positive visual images to do this? How do you feel and what is your thinking now about exercise and fitness? Spend a moment with your thoughts and as you do so find a word or a symbol that will remind you of this great feeling for the future.

Index

Bibliography

Adams, Jenni, *Relax and Unwind*, David & Charles, 1989

Garfield, Charles, A *Peak Performance*, Warner Books, 1984

Health Education Authority, *Physical Activity,* 1999

Health Education Authority, *Physical Activity Later in Life,* 1999

Health Education Authority, *What We Think,* 1999

Her Majesty's Stationery Office, *The Allied Dunbar Fitness Survey,* 1992

Hodges, Jeffery D., *Champion Thoughts, Champion Feelings* Sports Mind
    International Institute for Human Performance, 1998

Hodges, Jeffery D., *Sports Mind*, Sports Mind International Institute for
    Human Performance Research, 1999

Knight, Sue, *NLP at Work*, Nicholas Brealey Publishing, 1995

McArdle, William D., Katch, Frank I., Katch, Victor L., *Exercise Physiology,*
    Williams & Wilkins Publishers, 1996

McDermott, Ian and O'Connor, J., *Principles of NLP,* Thorsons, 1996

Mitchell, Laura, *Simple Relaxation,* John Murray Publishers Ltd, 1977

Palmer, Roy, *The Performance Paradox*, Delany & Smith, 2001

Tebbetts, Charles, *Hypnosis and Other Mind Expanding Techniques,*
Westwood Publishing Company Inc., 1987

YMCA, *Exercise and Fitness Knowledge*

Acknowledgements

I am thoroughly honoured to have had my 'think yourself' concept accepted by Cassell Illustrated and for the faith shown for my ability to write three books in a row. My thanks to Jackie Strachen and Mark Smith for that belief in the concept. Also to my agent Vicky McIvor for her encouragement and support. Many thanks to Victoria Alers-Hankey for all her help. Although this concept for encouraging the nation to get moving is mine alone it comes through knowledge that I have acquired over the years through my many different courses and of course my experience with clients. I most whole-heartedly want to thank Sports Psychologist Jeffery Hodges. BSC (AES) MSC for deepening my knowledge from his Sports Mind Course. I would recommend any fitness professional or NLP practitioner with an interest in sport to attend www.sportsmind.org.

I would also like to thank the Atkinson Ball College of Hypnotherapy and Iits training seminar for NLP. Thankyou to Michael Kaufmann Master Practitioner in NLP for his support. My grateful thanks to Bill Morton and the photographic team for the fabulous pictures and to Martyn Fletcher for the make up. Thanks also to the Leotard Company for providing the stunning outfits that enhance the visual aspect of this book. Thank you to The Fitness Network for lending the fitness equipment for this book. Lastly but by no means least of all, I would like to thank my friends and family for their support and encouragement and for putting up with me always working.